Praise for *Rituals*

"Personal, grounded rituals becor
steadiness within, no matter what happening
Allow Kori Hahn to guide you toward creating practices that
hold you every day."

— **Elena Brower**, bestselling author of *Practice You* and
Being You and founder of Essential Mentorship

"The ultimate go-to reference guide for ancient teachings
made modern. Here's to your more meaningful life!"

— **Emma Mildon**, bestselling author of
The Soul Searcher's Handbook and *Evolution of Goddess*

"*Rituals of the Soul* is a truly beautiful book. I felt an immediate connection to Kori Hahn and the way she takes you on
a journey toward living your most abundant, authentic life
through her story. Like Kori, I believe up-leveling your life is
available to anyone. That living in flow with your life rather
than against the current is within your reach. That in order
to unlock your soul purpose, you must tune in to your inner
wisdom and challenge yourself at every opportunity. As a
fellow yogi and travel lover, I can appreciate the pictures she
paints in each chapter. This guide to a modern and meaningful life will support you in clearing limiting blocks that stop
you from living in your flow and finding your soul's purpose."

— **Sophie Jaffe**, founder of Philosophie

"Kori Hahn's words are water for the dried desert flowers of
this world wishing mightily to open their petals and be born
again. This book contains eloquent and deep truths that the
world has needed to hear for a long time."

— **Janne Robinson**, CEO of This Is for the Women and
author of *This Is for the Women Who Don't Give a Fuck*

"This is the perfect book for intuitively connecting to the sacred rhythm of your life. With a deep understanding of both intuition and ritual, Kori Hahn masterfully guides you to create a unique personal practice for your soul's purpose. *Rituals of the Soul* shows you how to find not just *the* way but *your* way — one breath at a time."

— **Kim Chestney**, author of *Radical Intuition: A Revolutionary Guide to Using Your Inner Power*

Rituals
of the
Soul

Rituals
of the
Soul

**Using the 8 Ancient Principles of Yoga
to Create a Modern & Meaningful Life**

KORI HAHN

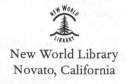

New World Library
Novato, California

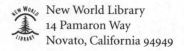 New World Library
14 Pamaron Way
Novato, California 94949

Text design by Tona Pearce Myers
Illustrations by Tracy Cunningham

Library of Congress Cataloging-in-Publication Data

Names: Hahn, Kori, author.
Title: Rituals of the soul : using the 8 ancient principles of yoga to create a modern & meaningful life / Kori Hahn.
Description: Novato, California : New World Library, 2021. | Includes bibliographical references. | Summary: "Yoga teacher, podcaster, and blogger Kori Hahn presents a new-age guide for harnessing the principles of yoga to manifest a better life. The book teaches readers how to develop simple, personalized rituals using techniques such as affirmations, breath work, meditation, journaling, and visualization" -- Provided by publisher.
Identifiers: LCCN 2021030111 (print) | LCCN 2021030112 (ebook) | ISBN 9781608687527 | ISBN 9781608687534 (epub)
Subjects: LCSH: Yoga. | Spiritual life. | Spirituality.
Classification: LCC B132.Y6 H245 2021 (print) | LCC B132.Y6 (ebook) | DDC 181/.45--dc23
LC record available at https://lccn.loc.gov/2021030111
LC ebook record available at https://lccn.loc.gov/2021030112

First printing, October 2021
ISBN 978-1-60868-752-7
Ebook ISBN 978-1-60868-753-4
Printed in Canada on 100% postconsumer-waste recycled paper

 New World Library is proud to be a Gold Certified Environmentally Responsible Publisher. Publisher certification awarded by Green Press Initiative.

10   9   8   7   6   5   4   3   2   1

Intuitive realization is the king of sciences, the royal secret, the peerless purifier, the essence of dharma (man's righteous duty); it is the first perception of truth — the imperishable enlightenment — attained through ways (of yoga) very easy to perform.

— THE BHAGAVAD GITA IX:02

Contents

Introduction

Only the dreamer knows the dream.

— CARL JUNG

I am a dreamer, and just as John Lennon said, I know I'm not the only one. Since I was a little girl, I have always found myself passionately pulled to try new things. In high school, I dreamed of playing the guitar like Sheryl Crow. In college, I imagined traveling the world with only a simple backpack. And now, in my late thirties, my heart yearns to feel as calm and cool as the Dalai Lama always appears to be.

Many people have told me that my dreams are a way of running away from my reality, and for years I considered this a truth, but now I realize that dreams are merely a fun way our soul gives us to learn our life lessons. Your dreams are illuminating the life path your soul wants you to take.

The reason you are here in your specific human body is to feel your dreams and act on them. From the moment of your conception, your soul picked you (and the skin you wear) because you are absolutely perfect for the purpose and mission your soul wants you to experience.

There are 7.6 billion other people here on Earth. Since most of us humans are designed fairly similarly, what makes us each truly authentic are our particular fiery passions and whatever it is that makes our hearts skip a beat. We all have unique things that make us tick, that bring us excitement and inspiration. For some people this may be music or writing; for others, it might be a particular sport or perhaps creating a successful career. There is no limit to the things we are passionate about. What do you do just because you love it?

This wild part of you that craves accomplishing certain things is your soul begging you to grow. If you feel that you were not born to spend 75 percent of your life working at a job you hate or staying in a marriage that keeps you bored or angry, this is your soul asking you for change. If you are looking for a sign to finally start making the changes you want to see in your life, perhaps that looking itself is the sign you need.

Every year, the bar-tailed godwit migrates from Alaska to New Zealand on a journey that takes approximately nine days, the longest known nonstop flight of any bird on the entire planet. Just like the godwit, every animal here on Earth is meant to take grand adventures that might at first feel daunting and scary but are such an important part of our life journey. The purpose of our human life is to commit to our soul's magnetic migrations — to listen for the guidance of our soul, our intuition, and then act on it.

In humans, this instinctive calling from within often comes to us in our dreams. Dreams offer us guidance along our personal migration route, just as the caribou, the whales, the butterflies, and many species of birds — including the godwit — have their own internal migration guidance system. Our individual journeys are as unique to us as the ridges on our thumbs.

You are born to be wild; this couldn't be more obvious. You are here to live out the wild adventures your soul is constantly calling you toward, because these heart passions guide you to grow and evolve in specific ways along your spiritual path.

What are your dreams? Do you know? If not, don't worry, I am here to help you realize and act on them.

Intuition

Dreams are just one of many ways intuition speaks to us. Our dreams often appear on the quietest of nights, like a northern star in a dark desert sky. At least, this is how my intuitive messages have come to me. When I stop all the doing and becoming in order to simply listen, in these moments my dreams always demand my attention.

The renowned Swiss psychiatrist Carl Jung defined intuition as "our perception via the unconscious" and went on to explain that perception using our senses — sight, hearing, taste, smell, and touch — is only a starting point. In fact, we bring forth ideas, images, possibilities, and/or ways out of a blocked situation by a process that is mostly unconscious. Scientifically, intuition is viewed as knowledge in the absence of analytical reasoning or logic.

Intuition is our way of perceiving the world through the lens of our soul, not from our mind or our expectations. Intuitive messages come from a place deeper in our consciousness than the thinking mind. You cannot think your way to an intuitive decision; intuition can be felt only through excitement, curiosity, and passion — your unexplainable urges. When a spark of a wild idea or a crazy dream comes to you and fills your mind with delight for what could be, you are receiving messages from your soul.

Our intuition is a soft-spoken, subtle voice whispering from the deepest, most subconscious place within. When we first start to tune in to it, intuition sounds remarkably faint, which is probably why so many people often ignore it. The more fluent we train ourselves to be in this language of soul whisperings, the louder and clearer it becomes.

In this book, I will share with you a system for hearing these whispers, through the ancient personal development path of yoga. You will learn not only how to hear your own innate intuition but how to identify what might be blocking you from following these messages. Hearing these whispers is the key to using your human life for the purpose your soul is asking of you. I hope to teach you how to do just that.

The Logical Path

Imagine being the bar-tailed godwit standing at the edge of the sea in Alaska, ready to take flight for New Zealand. How many logical thoughts would be going through your head, stopping you from taking that first leap of faith? I know my mind would be saying things like: "Oh, you little godwit, your wings are much too tiny for such a long and strenuous journey; it is much better for you to stay here, where it's sunny all day and the food is plentiful." But if the first godwits had listened to the logic of a human mind, those sweet little winged birds would be long extinct by now. The godwit likely would have stayed in Alaska, only to perish in a fruitless and frozen landscape.

One of the most significant differences between the birds and you is your ability to think intellectually. This is what makes living intuitively harder for us as humans. Intuition is not always logical. In fact, intuition is often anything but logical.

Humans tend to overthink our way out of intuitive decisions. Logic pulls us away from the wild, instinctive, innate form of perception and pulls us into the safe, easy, predictable. Logic keeps us fooled into staying in complacent situations, often telling us our dreams are silly, far-fetched, and unachievable. Logic prefers assurance and safety. Logic despises risk. And there are many times in my life when logic has kept me sitting on a shore that soon felt frozen and dead, rather than taking the gut-guided flight toward my dreams, just like the godwit.

Human life is meant to be a wild and carefree experience, where uncertainty and unpredictability are simply the reality of our existence. You were put in your body to live through amazing experiences, even if they at first appear to be overwhelming and intimidating.

Every modern-day spiritually seeking human wants to know their life's purpose. We want our lives (and even more so our suffering) to have some sort of greater meaning.

Ask yourself these questions: *Is my life a wild exploration, or does my life feel mundane and lack excitement? Is the life I am living based on logical reason and society's expectations, or am I doing exactly what makes my heart beat a little faster with passion and enthusiasm? If I listened more intently to what my heart wants, what would I be doing? What are my dreams, and why am I not living them at the moment?*

We are raised in a world full of societal expectations. You

go to school, meet a partner, buy a car and a house, get married, and possibly have children. If you do this and work hard, then you are a "good person." But where in this entire pre-drawn-up plan of my life is there room for me, my passions, my happiness, and my excitement?

We are trained our entire lives to do things logically, but the ancient gurus of yoga have always encouraged us to soften the mind's voice of logic in order to hear the whispers of our heart and soul, our intuition. The yogis have always understood that our soul's migration is found through our intuitive guidance, not through the logical. When we act on these intuitive urges, we connect to our ultimate purpose as a soul in a human body.

There is a big, beautiful purpose to your life, and in my experience, logic and science are not the keys to finding it. When we ignore intuition for whatever reasons, we are neglecting our soulful purpose. We sabotage any chances we have to feel the calming contentment that comes from walking our own unique path. We dismiss all the abundant possibilities we have to create a life that will lead to us feeling absolutely alive in each moment.

When we don't live the lives we were put on this Earth to live, feelings of emptiness and unease start to overwhelm our daily existence. In this situation, it is so easy for depression and anxiety to slip in. Deep unhappiness and unsettled feelings take over, because we are not aligning ourselves with the inner world we came here to bring forth.

Remember, you were born to be wild. And those inner whispers telling you to be even more wild are how your soul is guiding you. In this book, you will learn to move within, to find clarity on what your soul wants from you, and to put simple daily rituals in place to help make these dreams a reality. When you create the rituals for each step and diligently practice them, your life will become more soulful and exciting! Your life will become the creation of your dreams.

The Purpose of This Book

This book is a guide to soulful living, as explained by the world's greatest (and oldest) yogis. Its backbone is based on an ancient text, the Yoga Sutra of Patanjali. Compiled sometime between 500 BCE and 400 CE, it is a collection of 196 Sanskrit sutras (short precepts) on the theory and practice of yoga. Over the years since the scripts were discovered, many scholars, spiritual teachers, and yoga practitioners have continued to explain the sutras in ways that help us more deeply understand them and integrate them into our lives. I have translated some of the specific Sutras into my own words, as I feel they become easier for you to understand and remember this way. In those cases where I am sharing my own translation, it is indicated in the endnotes in the back of the book.

This book will teach you how to use yoga to connect with and start acting on your intuition. As explained in the old Sanskrit texts compiled by the wisest of yoga masters, this step-by-step system of spiritual growth and personal development is not based on religion but is more about finding your own inner truth through self-exploration and self-inquiry.

No matter what your religious or spiritual beliefs are, I believe you will find this book useful. If you don't know what your spiritual beliefs are or consider yourself an agnostic or an atheist, the system I will teach you can be incredibly helpful for discovering what spirituality actually means to you. This volume will offer you a broad understanding of yoga, not simply as a form of exercise or a tool for mental health, but as a means of soul revival and spiritual rejuvenation.

Most importantly, this book is meant to help you understand not just yoga but, through the process of experimenting with it, yourself.

I

The Intuitive Yogi

I am a little pencil in the hand of a writing God
who is sending a love letter to the world.

— MOTHER TERESA

It takes our entire life journey full of ups, downs, and side to sides to fully embody the deep soul experiences we were born as humans to be transformed by.

When I was twenty-one years old, my college boyfriend died suddenly and unexpectedly. The moment I heard the news, I fell to my knees in the parking lot outside my apartment and screamed at the top of my lungs, "*NO!*" The day my friend exhaled for the final time, my life began a very different course. I stayed awake night after night contemplating where his soul had gone and why I was still here, living.

A few months after his funeral, my poetry professor asked me if I would like to come to a yoga class she was teaching at the local gym. Thank God I said yes to her that day, because I found an amazing tool for healing my intense grief and growing into my truest, most authentic self.

In the beginning, I practiced yoga like most people do, a little movement combined with conscious breathing and perhaps a few meditations here and there. These practices most certainly made me feel better. I became a devoted student of the spiritual, at least when life became difficult — that was always when I dove in a little deeper. When things seemed to be flowing well, I carelessly floated through the practices.

I spent twenty years experimenting with different styles of yoga, types of meditation, and schools of theology. One day five years ago, while lying in bed after completing a yoga nidra meditation, I had an epiphany, a newfound perspective on yoga. Suddenly I realized that yoga is not just the hodgepodge of practices I had learned over the years but a ladder for helping us climb to our greatest selves — our soulful selves. I began to see the yoga system as a fully integrated eight-step process for connecting us to our soul's purpose.

I immediately started researching my ideas and gaining a larger understanding of the system as a whole, not just the parts I had always learned in yoga classes. Through that research, I found it most interesting that my copy of Patanjali's Yoga Sutras actually contains no pictures of postures whatsoever. In fact, in the whole big book there is only one simple line on using yoga as a movement practice, advising us to let our postures be comfortable and steady. All the other 196 aphorisms are focused on using the process of yoga as a personal growth tool, a guidance system for living. So I asked myself, "Why have I only been bobbing between the first two steps of the staircase when there are eight definitive steps listed for arriving to the temple of oneself?"

Yoga is a process, a system, a guide to returning home to yourself. When you start to see it that way, you stop focusing on the details of each step and start to notice the entirety of the stairway. And once you start to walk the stairway, you begin to understand the journey of the soul living within you.

Seven years ago, when I left an eight-year relationship and moved out of the beautiful home my partner and I had created together, I packed a small suitcase and drove a few hours into the mountains of Alaska. My destination was an off-the-grid, heavily weathered Mongolian-style yurt offered to me by a friend, far from the buzz of electricity and the free-flowing convenience of running water. For the first time in my life, I came to a full stop, liberated from distraction so that I could sit in nature and learn about myself.

I stayed in the woods for six long, dark Alaskan months, enjoying the isolation and quiet the place offered. The leaves turned golden yellow...then red...then brown...before a thick white blanket of snow covered them all. I watched the leaves and then the snow fall. I spent most of the daylight hours gathering firewood and skiing between the trees. Despite the fact that I had plenty of money to travel and explore, my soul was clearly asking me to spend this time here, off the grid, to simply listen to myself and learn to hear my intuition. During this period, I found out what it was I really wanted for myself and my life: I wanted to feel a deep sense of contentment and genuine happiness that I had never known before.

Most of my friends worried about me, thinking I had truly hit rock bottom. They would ask, "Kori, why did you leave your beautiful life, your loving partner, your comfortable cabin to live off the grid in a yurt?" I never really knew how to answer them, as I didn't completely understand myself at the time.

There were many moments when I questioned my sanity as well, especially when reminiscing about the warm, comfortable life I'd given up. To many it seemed I had had it all — love, safety, and comfort — but as hard as it was to explain to people, I had simply felt the urge to leave those things behind.

I spent a lot of time writing and drawing in my journal; many of those nights, tears streamed down my cheeks, smudging my ink drawings. But what no one in my life realized — what I didn't even realize at first — was that in order to see shooting stars, you must sit quietly staring at the sky. This was my time for stargazing.

While in hibernation that winter, I saw more stars than I had ever seen in my life. I practiced yoga to the crackling of my potbellied woodstove. I read inspiring books on travel and adventure. Most importantly, I listened to the messages as they rose up from inside me.

Those six months in the wilderness gave me the time and space I needed to take a deeper look into myself and understand what my intuition was asking from me. I continued my twenty-year yoga practice but stopped caring about the different styles and labels of yoga. I released myself from the often militaristic commitment to practice an hour of movement followed by thirty minutes of meditation, and I started doing any and all practices that I felt an urge to do, even if only for ten minutes. I learned to integrate yoga into my life no matter how little or how much time I had available for it. The benefits I started to receive from my practices grew exponentially.

In the spacious, still, and silent environment of Alaska that winter, I started hearing my dreams loudly. They were *yelling* at me. I recorded those messages in my journal. On one page, I made a list of twenty of the best surf towns in the world. On another page, there were quotes by Kurt Vonnegut and Clarissa Pinkola Estés about roaming and traveling. As I looked back through the pages of my journal a few months later, the black ink on those white pages made it very clear that what I really wanted was to travel and learn to surf.

It sounds so simple — traveling somewhere to surf — but that decision was the first step toward the most significant transformation of my life. It came to me as a dream, seemingly meaningless and silly, but I can assure you it changed the trajectory of how I was living, where I was living, the jobs I was doing, and the reality I was choosing to live in.

At the time, it felt unbelievably scary. I felt like I was leaving everything behind — my home, relationship, friendships, immense comfort, and a certain level of predictability — but what I ultimately left in Alaska was the part of me that had never had the courage to go after my wild and crazy soul dreams. I didn't yet know anything about how to manifest, but the only thing that made me excited to wake up every morning was that silly urge to dance upon the sea. Every time I saw a photograph of a longboard surfer girl, my heart raced with excitement. I knew I had to follow that tingle.

I might have left Alaska to surf, but eventually, that journey also led me to start my own business, meet someone special, have a child, write a book, travel the world, and settle into a new life in Sri Lanka. The conscious decision I made to follow that first surfing dream allowed other dreams to unfold. For the first time in my entire life I felt I was exactly where I was meant to be, living the purpose of my soul with a calm, settled contentment.

Through the same spacious calm that allowed me to hear my dreams, I started having epiphanies of a new and fresh approach to the ancient practice of yoga, making it incredibly simple and easy to commit to. I was able to embody the benefits I had yearned to receive from the practice for all those years! But more than that, I was able to use yoga to help me integrate what I wanted into my life and create it anew.

The first thing I did was to follow my intuition and start choosing my yoga practices on the basis of my intention — what I wanted to feel. I found that I did not need to perform every yoga pose, technique, and system. In fact, I discovered more power and efficiency by selecting a few practices and turning them into daily rituals. By committing to a few simple yogic rituals each and every day, I was able to manifest certain feelings within myself, like peace and calm or health and happiness. From this newfound understanding of yoga, I could then sit back and watch the rituals transform my entire life without all the stressful yearning and impatient craving I had experienced before. I started to see the results of the practice too as an embodiment of my intention.

This is the method at the core of this book. Through this simplified, ritualistic way of practicing yoga, you will know why you are practicing. You infuse first your entire yoga practice and then your entire life with intention, giving it purpose and meaning. You simply plug yourself in to the soul behind the wall.

The more I calmed my nervous system, cleared out the clutter of my life, and stopped to listen to my body on a subtle level, the more I realized that my yoga rituals were guiding me into my subconscious soul, teaching me how to live from the orb of feelings within.

I learned to fully relax on a subconscious level by using meditation. I learned to break through deeply rooted limiting beliefs by repeating simple "I am" affirmations on a daily basis.

I learned to pray by studying the stars with astrology and singing sacred chants to Hindu deities and patiently waiting for miracles to return to me.

Then, I began to experiment with using my simple little yoga rituals to manifest big, audacious, crazy ideas. At first, I followed dreams to acquire "stuff" and increase my material wealth by focusing on business, productivity, and success. While I was proud of what I managed to create for myself over these years, I found I was not happier or even content.

When I took the time to make sure my dreams were based on an idea of building a life of deeper meaning, I started creating less from a wound of worthlessness and more from a place of pure curiosity, with no expectation of what might come. I learned that when we surrender our days to doing more of what the soul wants, our life path feels more aligned and authentic. In my own experiments over the years, I found a way to use yoga as a ladder with which I could climb out of my deepest and darkest holes and start to touch the stars I wished upon.

The entire system of yoga is designed to help you heal your heart and your body and connect into your soul. You can use this ancient system to find your way when the grief, heartbreak, and hopelessness that appear in all of our journeys make you feel the lights have gone off completely.

Oftentimes our greatest creative moments and spiritual transformations emerge from our darkest of hours. In this book, we will journey through eight stages to help you get from where you currently are to where you hope to be.

I didn't create the eight-step strategy that I will reveal here. It is based on the teachings of the ancient yogis as explained in Patanjali's Yoga Sutras. These renowned sacred texts are often referred to collectively as "The Bible of Yoga," but they aren't the easiest material to read and are even harder to navigate as a guide for practical use. Often, the concepts are misunderstood, and the meaning of each sutra is sometimes lost in the translation of the ancient Sanskrit.

Nevertheless, the Yoga Sutras are just as renowned for their powerful guidance today as they were back then. To make them more accessible to you, however, I will share my own experiences and interpretations of each of the eight main principles of yoga.

You need to discover your soul's path, and that path is anything but logical. It's full of wild, sometimes downright intimidating decisions. So you need a strategy. Luckily, the yogis offer one: *the eight steps of yoga*. I will show you how to take all of their empowering and spiritually connecting concepts and integrate them into your everyday life through simple practices. You will create your own rituals for your own soul. The best thing about this book is that you can do this!

A Brief Introduction to Yoga

For thousands of years, people have asked the spiritual masters for help and guidance through the most challenging aspects of their lives. Over time, the yogis developed a step-by-step system that they found could be used by anyone and everyone to help them with their struggles. These spiritually developed mentors and teachers would look at their disciples and see which skills it would most benefit them to develop. Then they would give them practices for embodying those skills, like a spiritual prescription.

Yoga teaches you to gaze into yourself softly, quietly, and vulnerably so that you can hear what your soul is asking from you. Perhaps this is to build confidence, cultivate happiness, create spiritual connection, or follow a passion. When you hear your soul's messages and make an intention to embody them through certain practices, you create more moments of these feelings each and every day.

While the words of this book are very much my own, the system I have based it on is directly derived from the yogic scriptures, which lay out the details of this personal development science. Through the years many people have passionately experimented with this system, interpreting it for us and sharing their own examples of how the process has benefited them. I am lucky to have collected my own manifestation experiments using this eight-step system, which have proved to me just how efficient and powerful the yogis' method is for creating profound results in my life.

Paramahansa Yogananda, the renowned Indian yoga teacher who is credited with bringing yoga to the West, said, "A yogi engages himself in a definite, step-by-step procedure by which the body and mind are disciplined, and the soul liberated." Quite simply, the eight-step yoga system, this "step-by-step procedure," looks like this:

The Rules and Virtues of a Spiritual Being

1. The rules: *yamas*
2. The virtues: *niyamas*

Developing Your Intuition

3. Creating space: *asana*
4. Becoming mindful: *pranayama*
5. Developing awareness: *pratyahara*

Acting on Your Intuition

6. Unblocking and overcoming challenges: *dharana*
7. Believing and trusting: *dhyana*

Manifesting Your Dreams

8. Manifesting: *samadhi*

In the chapters that follow, you will become familiar with each of these steps and comprehend the big picture of yoga. By understanding, in a modern-day context, these eight concepts and the practices that help you cultivate them within yourself, you can use the steps to achieve a "soul liberated," as Yogananda explained. You learn to manifest your dreams, no matter what those dreams are.

Through the beautiful lessons offered to us by the most developed yoga scholars of the past, you discover how to live in harmony and alignment with the outside world. When you apply the concepts and regularly take moments to embody them, you start to feel the world around you lifting you up, rather than breaking you down. In an instant, you feel that you aren't dragging your feet to work every day but levitating (as the yogis would say) your way there. You have a sense of floating along life's path, and this feels like freedom.

As you use this book not only to intellectualize the process but to actually apply it each and every day through regular rituals, you will hear the pings of your intuition on a regular basis, opening the doors to your soul. When this happens, the yogis tell us we have no other option but to live through these pings.

Your Personalized Yogic Prescription

Both the ancient and modern yoga masters offer hundreds of yoga techniques and practices to help you along each of the eight steps. In asana, you will find many styles — Iyengar, yin, Ashtanga, vinyasa, Anusara, and hatha, just to name a few. The fifteenth-century manual the Hatha Yoga Pradipika delineates eight types of pranayama exercises, which can prepare you for thousands of types of meditation. From *vipassana* to chakra-clearing meditations, from Japanese Zen breath counting to Tibetan Buddhist *tonglen* meditations, you could spend your entire lifetime exploring different flavors.

Why are there so many yoga techniques and styles? Because yoga was first used primarily as a form of medicine. In the same way that you might go to the doctor to ask for help with a physical injury, many people in the past would go to the yoga gurus to ask for help for their ailments, physical, mental, and spiritual. In this book, I use the word *guru* to mean a person who understands a topic so thoroughly, they can teach their followers in a way that resonates and creates change. The gurus are the ones who give us prescriptions that work. To each of their followers, they appear to be wise in their topic of knowledge and efficient in their manner of teaching and advising them personally. My gurus' teachings could very well not resonate for you the same way they did for me. Similarly, you may have career gurus, health gurus, and spiritual gurus in your life who have really helped you find clarity in where you wanted to go and made it possible for you to get there, whereas their wisdom might not be meaningful for me.

Yoga has always been considered a form of therapy, a system full of practices for helping people find peace and harmony. In the past, the renowned yoga masters offered their followers a yogic prescription, usually unique to the patient. These prescriptions could have been specific meditations, or mantras to use, or perhaps even a simple stretch or movement to practice to release pain and tightness in the physical body. As you will see, the practices are endless. Learning when and how to use them gets slightly tricky, which is why a teacher or guru can be an invaluable asset.

In modern yoga practices, this teacher-student bond has been slightly diluted. In the West, yoga is mainly taught in commercial studios and, more recently, online. Unless you're practicing under the direct guidance of a yoga teacher who teaches in a very personal, soulful way, you might spend a lot of time learning techniques that don't resonate with you as an individual. Or perhaps the practices make you feel better, but you are not using them to their most powerful potential.

Yoga is meant to be a personal practice based on your unique needs. The more popularized physical form of yoga we see in the West today can help you learn the different practices available and gain skills for your toolbox, but to get the greatest effects, you need to create a practice specific to you. In the same way that your dreams and passions are personal, your yoga practices should be personalized.

If you don't feel intuitive or are generally indecisive, there are specific practices for connecting with a feeling-based magnetic compass that exists within you. If you do feel intuitive and clearly know your soul's needs, when your intuition sends you a dream, there are different practices that will guide you to manifest that reality for yourself. These practices become your soul rituals, revealing where you are yearning to go and navigating you there.

By creating a personalized set of rituals, you can move toward living a life of soul growth and eventually soul liberation. The Buddha became the Buddha in thirteen years. He did that one breath at a time. He made meditation his ritual, and he manifested enlightenment.

Big results come from baby steps. Birds migrate across oceans one flap of their wings at a time. In the same way, through your daily rituals, you will find clarity on what your dreams are and then you will manifest those dreams. With a bit of strategy and a heartfelt belief, you can manifest anything you want. Your dreams will begin to come true.

When you feel your life is aligning with the outer world more and more, you'll know the rituals are working. When you find more balance and harmony in your life than resistance, you'll know the rituals are creating an alchemy within you. When you start feeling a sense of contentment and purpose, you'll know you are connecting deeply with your soul. And you will only want to go deeper into yourself and further toward your dreams, because you have a step-by-step guide to help you do just that!

The Yogi's Rules: Yamas and Niyamas

Before we begin creating your own personalized set of powerful soul rituals, we must first go over ten fundamental guidelines to live by as advised by the yogis. The first two steps of yoga consist of five rules necessary for living a soulful life, called the *yamas*, and five virtues by which to guide your life, or *niyamas*. These fundamental guidelines resemble the Ten Commandments of the Judeo-Christian Bible and the Ten Virtues of Buddhism.

The yoga master B. K. S. Iyengar describes the yamas and

niyamas as "the golden keys to unlock the spiritual gates." While most of the rules and virtues are easy to check off your list, keep in mind that progressing along your spiritual path will be incredibly hard if you fail to adhere to these simple guidelines. And conversely, if you follow them, they will make it easier for you to receive the benefits of yoga. In particular, unlike the Ten Commandments, joy is a big part of the niyamas, which is exactly what your life purpose and manifesting the life of your dreams are all about. The niyamas guide you to find your personal path, discover what you love and what feels good to you, and trust in the universe to make things happen.

I want to mention these to you right away, because if you find it difficult to make a decision, you can return to the niyamas, or virtues, for help in making a soulful choice. We will explore the yamas and niyamas further throughout the course of the book, as well as the remaining six steps of yoga, but I urge you to at least familiarize yourself with them now. You may return to them later as needed.

Yamas: The Rules for a Spiritual Life

- Be kind. Don't harm: *ahimsa.*
- Be honest. Don't lie: *satya.*
- Don't steal: *asteya.*
- Respect your body and life as sacred: *brahmacharya.*
- Simplify. Minimize. Don't be wasteful: *aparigraha.*

Niyamas: The Virtues of a Spiritual Being

CLEANLINESS: *Saucha*

- Clean the body with exercise; clean your schedule to make more time; clean the mind with meditation.

- Clear out toxicity.
- Surround yourself with only the purest people, places, and environment.
- In India, there is a saying: "An unclean home leads to a messy mind." The things that make you feel calm and clear are the spiritual cleansing practices of saucha.

CONTENTMENT: *Santosha*

- If it makes you happy, do more of that.
- If it feels good to you, do it as often as you can.
- Do more of what makes your soul smile.
- Spend more time with the people who make you happy.
- The things you do that make you happy are the spiritual practices of santosha.

BURNING ENTHUSIASM: *Tapas*

- Follow the path that lights you up.
- Explore your curiosities.
- Follow your passions.
- Chase your dreams.
- The things that make you feel alive are the spiritual practices of tapas.

STUDY OF THE SELF: *Svadhyaya*

- Pursue the path of soul growth.
- Learn about your spirit.
- Experiment with what this life experience really means to you.
- Explore yourself through self-inquiry.
- The things that teach you about you are the practices of svadhyaya.

TRUST IN THE UNIVERSE: *Isvara Pranidhana*

- Energy and frequency are scientifically proven influential powers that surround us.
- Pray to God.
- Trust in a greater power.
- Understand the universe's immense powers in your life.
- The things that make you connect with your spirit are the practices of isvara pranidhana.

Return to the yamas and niyamas as often as you can; they are the most direct ways to connect to your soulful home within. Let the niyamas be a reminder of what to focus on and how to make decisions in your life. When you do, your life will start to fill with purity, contentment, passion, curiosity, and, above all else, trust.

Now you are ready to dive into the remaining six steps of the yogic system, which will offer you practices to support you in living this way.

When you follow this book as your own yellow brick road, it will take you to where you want to go. If you want to start by dreaming small, so be it. But if you dare, dream big.

The Yogic Path from Dreaming to Enlightenment

Take a second now to think of a dream that has come true in your life. What began as a flicker of inspiration, a shooting star of an idea, and became manifested into your reality?

If you haven't had that experience yet, don't worry — you will.

The journey you take from dreaming to manifesting is how you grow your soul. It's how you are guided to your life purpose. It's how you become your most authentic self, your soulful self.

A few strong manifestation moments for me are the day I completed my first vipassana meditation, when I became a certified boat captain, when I led my first yoga retreat, and the first time I sent my published book to someone to read. As I look back on my life, these manifestation moments stand out as the times when I felt my proudest and most purposeful because I had worked hard to make them a reality, determined and unshakable in my conviction. Then, they had happened!

Regardless of how big or small your dream may feel to you or how long you've been hoping for it to manifest, when it does, your dream will become your reality. You might feel a sense of soul contentment and satisfaction, of purpose and determination. You may experience deep peace in these moments, as I have, because you feel a connection to spirit, the sacred, and your soul like never before.

As you practice manifesting moments, you will learn to manifest on a much bigger scale, in cycles. It's like stepping into bigger and bigger shoes each time you do it. This is how you move toward the ultimate goals of your soul: enlightenment, liberation, and soul freedom.

Know that your soul has a very big mission for you. It may take many rounds of dreaming and manifesting to fully understand and implement this soul science into your life. The cycle of manifestation is the soul's way of magnetizing you toward more truth and freedom in each and every round. Once you understand how the process works, you will become increasingly efficient at it. And, more importantly, you will find more and more peace in the journey with every cycle you pass through.

Every dream you manifest will inspire you to manifest another. You will become more confident and feel more worthy as you reach for more ambitious dreams.

Just as with everything else, practice makes perfect. We can only baby-step our way through this practice, dropping little rituals into our day to create new habits in our lives. As you practice and refine your rituals over time, using different dreams and feelings as your objects of manifestation, you will grow more experienced in the eight steps of the cycle, preparing yourself for the greatest dream of all: soul liberation. Eventually, this method for manifesting will feel natural to you. You won't need this book anymore; the eight steps will just become your innate art of living.

The dreaming I speak of here isn't clingy or desperate; it simply consists of learning to use passion and soul-sent messages to guide you along your spiritual path. You should be in no hurry or rush to see the results, although we all naturally tend to want to in the beginning. We simply are using our dreams as objects of experimentation to get to know ourselves and how our own consciousness, subconsciousness, and spirituality function.

The migration of the monarch butterfly explains this cycle well — this concept of cycling our way to our enlightenment, liberation, and soul freedom. One single migration, which goes from the southern Canadian mountains to the hills of central Mexico, takes the monarch butterfly four different generations to make. Four cycles of life, death, and rebirth happen in the journey from point A to point B.

Along the monarch migration route, the first three generations of butterflies live their lives striving to reach the treetops of Michoacán, but they never do. It is only with the help

of these ancestral butterflies that the fourth butterfly genera-
tion finally arrives at its destination in middle Mexico. These
delicate winged creatures never lose focus over the 5,000-
kilometer journey; their instinctive navigation system keeps
them moving in the direction they are meant to go, typically
traveling fifty to a hundred miles a day.

Once again, baby steps create big results. The monarch
butterflies' journey is neither short nor easy, and your journey won't be either. It takes two months for the tiny butterflies
to complete their entire migration journey, the equivalent of
300 human years. Your own soul growth relies on the momentum of every intuitive spark you chase in the same cyclical life
pattern of the monarch to get you to where your soul is determined to go.

Humans grow spiritually in steps and stages, one passionate
push at a time, possibly over many lifetimes. Like the monarchs, we are born exactly where we belong in this life to continue pursuing our spiritual evolution. You don't know how
many dreams it will require or how long it will take you to get
there, but you are working toward something incredibly important — your soul's ultimate freedom.

And if you ever get the chance to go to those sacred hilltops
in Michoacán to see the final resting place for all the millions
of monarchs who made it back to their soul home, it is an absolutely incredible sight to see, trees heavily weighted down
and the ground completely carpeted in a thick blanket of butterfly wings. It is the sort of sight that makes you believe there's
a God. I imagine this must be a bit of what it is like when all of
our human souls move into the final liberation phase. It will be
magical, just like the arrival of the monarchs.

Yoga is one of the greatest tools I have encountered for spiritual evolution because it teaches us how to connect with our soul. We learn how to read the road map to our dreams — how to see all the possible routes available to us to get there — and then, like the monarch, we simply start flapping along.

2

Creating Space

*When you tidy your space completely, you transform the scenery.
The change is so profound that you feel as if you are
living in a totally different world.*

— Marie Kondo

After the brief mention of the rules and virtues, creating space is the first step the yogis gave us to becoming more intuitive. This is the perfect place for everyone to begin their journey. You must create more space in your life by minimizing busyness. Then you can better feel the soft, subtle messages of the soul.

How often do you notice shooting stars when you are intensely working? Or binge-watching Netflix? Or hiding away? You see shooting stars only when you stop and look up at the spacious sky above you. The best observatories in the world are all in remote, clear settings — places like the summit of Mauna Kea volcano in Maui, the Atacama Desert in northern Chile, the frozen plains of Wisconsin, and the South Pole in Antarctica.

Spaciousness is also within. How often do you check in with your body or your emotions and truly notice how you feel? How often do you stop and relax enough to let resistances and tension flow out of you? How often do you simply take the space to stop and lie down?

Think of it this way: you can go to France and spend your entire vacation sightseeing. You can climb to the top of the Eiffel Tower and stroll through the Louvre. But you will never truly feel like you are in France until you sit at a little streetside café sipping an espresso in a tiny cup.

Similarly, feeling into yourself requires taking a peaceful moment to rest, look at the space that lives within, and expand it. Creating space is about pausing amid the action and then taking the time to feel the ambience. This is what creates the full "*Oui, oui*, I am actually in France" experience. The same is true of visiting your inner space.

Although I already shared with you how I created space one crucial winter in Alaska, I actually spent twelve years of my life in the state, learning to settle into my own spaciousness. When I arrived there, it felt like an entirely different world from where I had grown up in big-city Texas.

The first two summers, I worked in Native villages so remote I had to take a tiny four-seater Cessna to get there. I spent most of the bright and long summer days sitting on the banks of slow-moving rivers or teaching children to swim in calm ocean coves. I learned how to spend my days simply being exactly where I was.

I fell head over heels in love with the vastly spacious, silent world I discovered. Upon my return to the small ski town I called home for most of my years in Alaska, I continued to move deeper into an ascetic, slow lifestyle. Over the years I found myself yearning to leave behind the comforts of electricity, running water, and concrete roads for a more off-the-beaten-track existence.

Despite what many might think, my off-the-grid life didn't mean I had ample opportunities to sit around and meditate like a monk in a Himalayan cave. I hauled water in large five-gallon jugs, shoveled pathways through the snow, and chopped a whole lot of firewood for most of the year. But while I did these things, I found a lot of time to hear the thoughts of my mind and distinguish them from the whispers of my soul.

In this period of quiet stillness, I found the space I needed to reevaluate what was important to me. I left behind the partying lifestyle so many of my college friends were living and many of the pressures society had ingrained in me. Rather than work my way up the corporate ladders of America, I chose to hike up mountains instead. I traded the big stores with unlimited shopping options for a life of hunting and gathering my own foods. Ultimately, I left the busyness.

Once all the firewood was chopped and the cooking was done (as you can imagine, there were no restaurants nearby), I would make a cup of tea and read the books I had selected for the month, usually borrowed from a friend or library, but always handpicked to nurture the current curiosities bubbling up from within me. I would paint and write simply because I enjoyed those things. This is how spaciousness gives us the room we need to grow our soul. It allows us to listen to the voice within, feel for our passions, and spend time nurturing them.

The more space you can create in your life, the more room you make for newness. Whether the newness you desire is to manifest one particular thing or to cultivate a specific feeling in yourself, you still need to open the space for that thing or feeling to grow. By making more time, more room, and more stillness, you cultivate an open environment that's perfect for your intuition to move into.

Busyness, stress, and tension are the first layers of blockages between you and the subtle sensations of your intuition. When it comes to manifesting your dreams, think of them as a garden. Nothing grows through rock-hard tension. Your intuition, which is the voice of your soul, is always speaking to you, but when your overscheduled mind and body are distracted and tense, you are unable to hear it.

The most fertile gardens in the world all have airy soil, abundant light, and plenty of oxygen. This is exactly the kind of environment you must create for yourself. Only then can your intuition seep through the cracks and pool toward the surface.

Space is a vessel for new creations to grow within. By learning to release tension, trauma, and stagnation, you create space in the body and mind. The body and mind naturally grow calm through this process. As you learn to eliminate what you don't particularly love about your life, you start to clearly see what you want to fill the newfound space with. Perhaps you exchange the busyness for more peace? Perhaps you spend less time doing what you think you should in order to prioritize more time doing what you love? Perhaps you realize how simplifying your life allows you to focus on diving into your passions and dreams?

In fact, simplification is one of the yogi's rules for living: aparigraha, the virtue of nonpossessiveness, nongrasping, or nongreediness and stripping one's life down to only what is necessary. In this space you will experience instantaneous impressions, like magnetizations, pulling you closer to particular places, ideas, and people. Intuitive sparks and heart pings will guide you toward a life you failed to even see before. The simpler your life, the easier these impressions are to feel.

"Creating space" is another term for letting go, and letting go happens in a few different ways. Sometimes, in relationships, people choose to let us go; and other times, we choose to walk away. In either scenario, we create space.

Grief is the biggest, most painful form of letting go. As you inevitably live through grief, loss, and heartbreaks, you will likely be reminded time and again of how soft and vulnerable your heart is. You may feel pain in your chest and fold your shoulders in to protect it. You may bow your head in defeat to the pain because it hurts too much to stay open and look ahead. We often avoid what is difficult to face, but just remember that in facing difficult situations, you are allowing your soul to grow. Many times, you must let go of something because it's the natural journey your soul wants your life to take. By staying soft, open, and vulnerable in these moments, you amplify your ability to create space. And, in turn, this space allows you reoccurring opportunities to heal.

Sometimes we have to stop being habitually busy in order to learn how to be habitually calm and spacious. To create more space in your life, you will first have to learn to let go of things that are sucking your energy. We must constantly return back to this process of letting go because it's part of the natural cycle of life, whether you like it or not.

People deal with painful emotions in one of two ways. They either allow a hard, protective, defensive shield to develop around their heart, or they keep their hearts soft and open, staying vulnerable and constantly expanding into what they are here to learn. The latter is the path of healing, personal development, and soul freedom.

The best thing you can do to live more connected to your heart and soul is to soften what has grown hard and make a conscious intention to create space whenever you feel resistance and tension. Make an intention to open when you want to close off. Stay soft and vulnerable even though the emotions moving through you are hard and overwhelming.

Creating space guides you to let go. It is the first step to listening to your intuition and viewing life like a vast, open canvas to paint your dreams upon. If you aren't sure what "creating space" truly means or how it feels, don't worry. I will share practices to help you start doing this. But it is important for you to understand the intention behind the practices first.

Postures

Asana, meaning "postures," is the third step of yoga. In the West, we tend to think of postures as something we do in yoga class when our teacher instructs us to form our body into a particular shape that might have some degree of difficulty for us. But I believe that traditionally yogis were simply talking about observing the various postures we naturally form with our bodies throughout the course of our days, whether sitting at work, lying down, or standing. The yogis guided us to look at our physical body as a lens through which to ask ourselves the questions: Is there tension? Am I comfortable? Do I feel tightness? Where can I create more space in my life? How can I feel more grounded, steady, and spacious?

This stage of yoga is actually much simpler than the modern world of yoga makes it out to be. It is described in one simple sutra of the nearly 200 written: "*Sthira sukham asanam*," meaning "[a position that is] steady and comfort[able]." The yogis specifically instructed us to create postures that are steady and comfortable every day. By doing this, you naturally create space in your mind and body. Take a look at all of the postures you practice in a day, such as sitting at your computer, walking the dog, eating dinner, and lying in bed. You will begin to see where you can integrate more space into your physical body and also where space seems to be limited in your daily schedule.

Start by reviewing your daily schedule. How busy or distracted is your mind on a regular basis? How tight or tense is your body in each specific posture you habitually take? How cluttered are the spaces where you live and work? You may be able to create more space in each of these areas of your life one by one. Don't overthink all this; try to let it be easy.

In Marie Kondo's bestselling book *The Life-Changing Magic of Tidying Up*, she guides readers to declutter as a way of creating more peace and harmony in their lives. The basis of Kondo's book is that you should focus on each thing in your life, one at a time, and ask, "Does this bring me joy?" Through the process of decluttering, you simplify your surroundings so they hold only things you genuinely love. Creating space in your mind and body is much the same; practicing fewer tension-filled postures throughout your day is about releasing what isn't bringing you joy in order to fill the space with what does.

As you practice creating a little extra space each and every day, you will build a habitual, subconscious pattern, something that you naturally do without thinking about it. As you cultivate more and more space, you will be better able to feel into your intuition to hear the messages of your soul awakening you to your soulful purpose.

EXERCISE: *Where in Your Life Do You Need More Space?*

It is not possible to create space in your life until you understand which activities and habits are making your life feel cluttered and busy. In the following exercise, I offer a list of questions for you to ask yourself in your journal. I encourage you to create a little mental space after writing down each question to simply observe what your intuition might be messaging to you. Some answers might come through loud and clear in an instant, and others might come slowly and subtly over time.

Also leave a little extra room (pun intended) after each answer so you can add more later. Come back to the questions again and again. Leave a little space not just in your journal but in your daily life for the answers to pop up. This is the entire point of this step of yoga, to create more space for anything and everything to arise. Simply start being aware of all the things you do and the postures you make and how these activities make you feel.

Carry the questions around with you throughout your day for a week or more, jotting down what you notice about your body and your daily schedule. Continue expanding on your answers until you have a complete image of what in your life needs to be more spacious and joyful. By focusing your awareness on what isn't working in your life and making an intention to let those things go, you create space for the things you really want to grow into.

Read each of the questions, sit with it for a few minutes in silence, and then write down any answers that appear to you:

1. How can I create more free time each day?
2. Where am I wasting or losing time?
3. What am I doing that doesn't bring me joy?
4. Where do I feel tight in my body?
5. Where do I hold tension?
6. Am I spending a lot of time during my day doing something I really dislike?
7. Am I easily distracted?
8. Does my environment bring me joy or stress?
9. Is there something that is sucking the energy out of my day?
10. How can I create more space in my life?

Creating Space in the Body

Let's talk a bit more about all the body postures you make in a day and how to create space specifically in the body. B.K.S. Iyengar describes this step of the yoga system as a process of "developing such an intense sensitivity that each pose of the skin acts as an inner eye." (He goes on to explain this step of asana as a stage of asking ourselves, "What am I doing?" and "Why am I doing it?")

To create space in the body, simply focus on how each part of the body is feeling, part by part. When you are drawn to an area that feels tense or tight, you can then start to create space in this particular region by softening in a way that releases tension. In other words, let your movements be guided by how you feel and how you want to feel.

Do you feel tension in your neck and shoulders, for example? The way you hold your shoulders indicates how protective you are of your heart. People are often more protective of their hearts when they carry memories of heartache and grief. If your shoulders fall inward, protecting and shielding your chest, you have an opportunity to open and expand the heart, making it more accessible. This is how you can create space in this area and open yourself up to more love.

Do you notice tightness around your hips? The hips are another place in which many people, especially women, tend to hold intense emotions. The tightness in your hips can happen when you have a fear of moving forward in your life. Our hips carry the weight of our entire upper body, including all the thoughts of the mind and pains of the heart. Our hips take the majority of our body and all the stories we hold within it and decide how that affects our ability to move forward. When we place our awareness in the hips and focus on creating space here, life starts to flow with more ease.

Creating space might mean breathing through the resistance and tightness that you have developed through habitual ways of dealing with subconscious traumas and emotions. If you have a regular yoga practice, try to begin each session by scanning your body and making a mental note of where you feel tension. Let your movement practice be motivated by this intuitive realization. Where you find tension and resistance, focus your energy on creating more space there. Breathe into this area as you open it, and feel little victories breaking through.

One common problem for most of us modern-day yogis is that we often work on computers, which may lead to neck and shoulder tightness on a regular basis. If this is true for you, start to integrate more space and softness into this area of the body by taking five-minute shoulder relaxation breaks several times during your screen-focused work sessions.

Your asana practice does not need to take an hour — in fact, it might take just a few minutes and consist of only one or two poses each day — but let this valuable time be focused on where you need it most. Think in terms of "How can I make myself more spacious right now?" and "What needs releasing?," and soon you will start unlocking the outer cages of your body, which keep your soul locked within. By creating more space, by making yourself more "steady and comfortable," as the ancient yogis advised, you allow your soul to live openly in every part of you.

Asanas to Create Space

If you already have a yoga practice or want to begin one, you might be interested in particular postures that help you create space. I suggest going to five yoga classes and writing down which postures give you a warm, open, expanded, glowing feeling. Refer to this list and stick with these for a little while. Your list of favored postures will grow over time, as will the space in your body.

To get you started, here are a few suggested postures for particular areas of the body (see the next page for illustrations):

To open the heart: Supported Fish
To create space in the hips: Dragon, Happy Baby
To create space in the thoughts: Child's Pose
To increase relaxation: Shavasana
To engage in flow and flushing movement: Sun Salutations

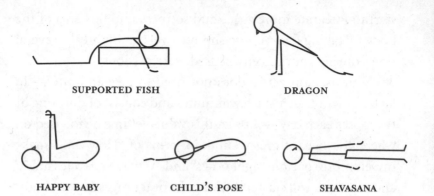

SUPPORTED FISH   DRAGON

HAPPY BABY   CHILD'S POSE   SHAVASANA

SUN SALUTATIONS

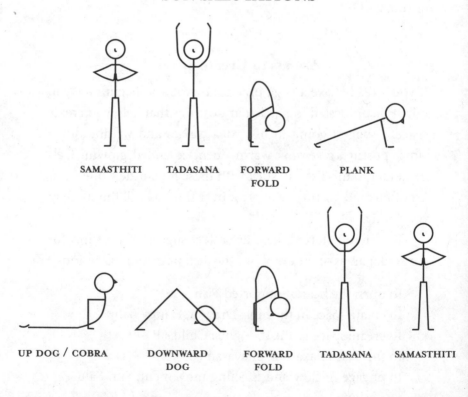

SAMASTHITI   TADASANA   FORWARD   PLANK
                                        FOLD

UP DOG / COBRA   DOWNWARD   FORWARD   TADASANA   SAMASTHITI
                          DOG   FOLD

Creating Space in the Mind

For nearly one year, I performed asana — physical posture practices — with the pure intention of tuning in to my intuition. With this goal in mind, my yoga practice morphed into long sessions of lying in Shavasana, flat on the ground like a corpse (the Sanskrit meaning of *shavasana*). When I lay on my back with my eyes closed, facing toward the sky, I was able to fully relax and stop doing. It was like taking a trip out to the remote villages in Alaska and just simply being with what was. When I did this, I could feel my intuition bubbling to the surface with more ease.

I stopped performing all the ups and downs you typically see in most modern-day yoga classes. I found these one-posture yoga sessions allowed me to reduce my internal clutter and release my habitual tendency to do more (as there is always more to do in the thinking mind). Now, I simply stop and lie down. Most days, nearly 50 percent of my yoga practice is simply stopping — doing less and relaxing more.

Does your mind feel busy or tense? Deep relaxation is one of the greatest ways to create space in the mind, the body, and therefore the heart, too. Most of the epiphanies in my life have come to me while relaxing comfortably on my back. That is why now it has become a ritual I try to return to daily, for a few minutes when I wake up, when putting my son to bed, and before going to sleep myself.

I encourage you to explore and be curiously drawn to the ways you are filling the space of your body. When you find an area you are intuitively called to let go in, find a way to make the body comfortable and steady. There is no right or wrong in this experiment; there is only learning.

Creating Space from the Heart

Yoga does not strictly need to be performed on a yoga mat. Anything that brings you joy and relaxation also creates space. If you are performing an action because you're passionate about it, there is no doubt that it's a catalyst for creating space within you.

I can assure you that for me, surfing is a powerful form of meditation, a helpful tool for letting go and decluttering the mind, and a source of immense joy. So I surf often. My grandmother might say that knitting brings her joy, and my mother would credit tennis! If something makes you happy, do it more often. If you feel you are creating space when you are on a tennis court, in the ocean, on a dance floor, or crocheting on a couch, do more of it. That too is yoga!

The Spaciousness Rituals

Creating rituals is one way to move toward the changes you would like to see in your life. Rituals build a bridge from where you are now to where you want to be. They don't have to be formal or difficult to create. A ritual is simply something you commit to doing for yourself on a regular basis. It can be as simple as taking time to create space for your body and mind by relaxing. But by calling it a ritual, you give that time the importance, respect, and reverence it deserves.

In his book *The Heart of Yoga*, the modern-day yoga teacher T.K.V. Desikachar, the son of a famous yoga guru, refers to the construction of a yoga sequence as *vinyasa krama*. *Vinyasa krama* means "in a special way [*vi*] to place [*nyasa*] the steps [*krama*]." Whatever you choose for your ritual is, in a very real way, your own yoga sequence.

In the following section, I will guide you in building your own vinyasa krama, or yoga sequence, for creating more space in exactly the ways you need. These space rituals are one of three daily practices (the other two being mindfulness and awareness) that are imperative for you to do in order to learn how to feel and hear your intuition with clarity. Let your yoga session each day be the special baby steps to which you're committing. These rituals will start to become your personalized strategy for soul growth and life creation.

Create Your Spaciousness Rituals:
Vinyasa Krama

There are a few primary considerations to keep in mind when creating your spaciousness rituals.

Time. How much time can you commit to your rituals without struggling? Remember, these are the first steps for manifesting your dreams, and as such, they are important. Still, you also need to be realistic about what you are going to accomplish and how long it will take. Once you know exactly how much time you can dedicate to your spaciousness rituals, you're ready to curate them.

Posture. Be mindful of every posture that you assume for an extended amount of time throughout the course of your day, whether sitting, standing, bending, or any other activity in which you regularly engage. Ask yourself whether each posture is creating spaciousness or tension. Minimize the specific postures that you find create tightness, busyness, or distraction, and begin swapping them out for more relaxing, calming, opening positions.

Is there something physical that you can do every day to

create more space? Many people feel more peaceful when exercising daily, possibly because exercise takes their mind off pressures and creates more oxygen in the body. Some Buddhists meditate because it creates a more spacious feeling in the mind. As I mentioned, I personally love to surf because it keeps me focused on the spaciousness and movement of the ocean and my physical posture. Take some time now to find out which postures resonate the most with you.

Relaxation. The more you relax, the more space you create. Imagine how you would feel if you committed to getting a massage once a week, or taking a bubble bath, or simply floating in the ocean. If you don't have a relaxation ritual already, adopt one now. Again, it can be simple. Don't overthink it — do whatever helps you relax and create more space in your body and mind.

Love. By doing something you love each and every day, you nurture yourself. In fact, making the time to do more of what you love is the key to a happier life. If you aren't sure what you love to do, explore and try something new! If you love it, stick with it.

Intuition. When you read my words about creating more space, what jumps to mind? Perhaps something you've been avoiding? Maybe you immediately thought to yourself, "I need to take care of all the junk in the back of my car!" If so, get busy cleaning that trunk out, because the voice in your head was your soul asking you to do that, but then come back to this spacious stage of listening and keep building on it. Always continue returning to this space to hear the whispers of your intuition. Your intuition is always leading you to let go of something, so try to let this voice be your ultimate guide for creating your powerful space rituals.

EXERCISE: *Embodying Spaciousness*

I recommend that your rituals always be present in your daily routine. If you decide to integrate the teachings of this book in your life, start by creating rituals or a regular practice for generating the skills I discuss in these pages.

Begin by planning your first spaciousness ritual. You can always adjust and alter it later however you wish, but make some decisions now so that you set the intention of performing the ritual regularly to create more space in your life.

At first, set a specific time when you will perform your ritual, either daily or weekly — not because it is absolutely necessary to perform it at the same time every day, but because it makes it easier to stay consistent and turn the practice into a habit.

Write down your answers to the following questions:

1. What helps you feel more space in your mind, body, and environment?
2. Is there a message inside you encouraging you to create space in a certain way?
3. Is there a spacious place where you can conduct your ritual regularly?
4. How much time will you commit to for your ritual?
5. What postures (traditional yoga or just day-to-day postures) will you use to stay relaxed and create more space during your ritual?
6. What activities nurture the feeling of "me time"?
7. What activities that bring you joy and relaxation will you make a part of your ritual? To help you decide, think about what you absolutely love to do, what you would choose to do every day for the rest of your life

if you could, and what might bring a fiery excitement into your life.

8. What do you consider sacred? What objects would help you bring that sense of the sacred into your ritual? Candles? Crystals? A particular book?

3

Becoming Mindful

The breath is a wonder drug.

— KRISHNAMACHARYA

Mindfulness is the fourth step in the yoga system. This step is a powerful one for developing focus and concentration. Mindfulness teaches us to keep our mind fully present in this exact moment — not in the past or the future, but right here, in the now. To be alert, awake, and fully immersed in the present moment is what it means to be mindful. In fact, many Buddhists often refer to mindfulness as "single-pointed concentration," which is quite the opposite of the multitasking, busy monkey mind that society encourages us to live with. Pranayama exercises, which focus our awareness single-pointedly on our breath, are how we become skilled in mindfulness.

In our modern-day society, especially in the Western world, we are taught from an early age to plan ahead, to focus on our future, and to constantly build our lives to be bigger and better. With this air of productivity surrounding us, there is an energetic drive pushing us to "grow and become." This is the energy we are raised in, making it incredibly difficult for us to simply rest in the present moment and allow the mind to feel calm and at peace.

Many of us have picked up a belief that stillness is a waste of time. We think that if we are busy, we are important and using our lives purposefully, but this is one of our greatest misperceptions. Have you heard the saying "Time is sacred, so make the most of it?" There is a belief that we only have so much time here on Earth, so we should rush to do all the things we want. Ironically, when we embody this belief, we end up wasting most of our time incessantly doing, rather than simply being.

In the past ten years, through the development and widespread use of smartphones, we have become habitually busy by spending an overwhelming amount of time online, searching, scrolling, posting, capturing, and connecting through social media. Most of you probably know by now that our phones are one of our greatest distractions, taking us away from what is happening in our more real and honest reality.

By developing your ability to stay mindful, you learn to focus on what is happening right now, in this present moment. As we start to integrate mindfulness into our lives, we realize that all the thoughts, emotions, and sensations moving through us are something separate and unattached to our mind. When we learn how to sit in the now and observe our thoughts, emotions, and sensations constantly arising and passing away, we start to understand their natural flow. We learn not to react to certain thoughts, not to focus on certain emotions; instead, we retrain the mind to rest in the space that allows all these sensations to flow through.

An overactive thinking mind is one of our greatest blockages to being great listeners, to others as well as to ourselves. In order to hear the messages of your soul, you must learn to listen. And without a strong intention to consistently bring your thinking mind back to this present moment, you don't hear important things people say, because the chatter in your head is distracting you from being fully engaged with the people you are interacting with. When you start to feel the harmony and balance that comes with a regular mindfulness practice, you will see immense opportunities waiting for you each and every day.

Throughout this book, I am teaching you simply to listen to yourself. In each chapter, I explain how the concepts and practices the yogis offered us are tools for developing the skills you need to hear your intuition. At times the process might be uncomfortable, because you are changing lifelong habits of busyness and distraction.

In *A New Earth: Awakening to Your Life's Purpose*, the spiritual teacher and author Eckhart Tolle explains mindfulness this way: "Rather than being your thoughts and emotions, be the awareness behind them." The only way to learn this language of your soul and become fluent in it is to become habitually mindful. In other words, mindfulness is the nonnegotiable skill necessary to connect you with your soul's purpose. If you fail to develop this skill, all the other steps we will move into from here simply cannot happen. Only when you are mindfully aware of what is happening in your body in each moment can you truly know what your intuition is saying to you.

Life gives us thousands of choices and decisions to make each day. If you are not mindful and present in the now, you will be blind to all the little roads right there in front of you, which are waiting to take you where your soul wants you to go.

When you start to gain control of your mind, teaching it to focus single-pointedly, you gain a superpower ability to get things done. If you want to focus on the good in your life, it becomes much easier to focus on just that. Likewise, if your mind has a tendency to worry about the future and give you anxiety, you can minimize that reaction by simply staying in the present more fully. As you teach your mind to live in the present, you will start to find the natural peace that exists within you.

Meditation is the most popular practice for becoming more mindful. You begin by learning how to concentrate the mind. The most common objects to meditate on are the breath and the sensations of the physical body, because no matter where you are or what you are doing, your breath and your body will be there for you as tools. More importantly, you are learning to concentrate on what's happening within you right now, in each and every moment. Simply put, a mindfulness meditation practice is the process of concentrating on whatever is happening in this moment within the body and letting your awareness of everything else become quiet.

During your mindful meditation, when the mind runs away to the land of thoughts and daydreams, you simply need to bring it back to what is actually happening now within your body. You notice: the body is breathing, and the heart is beating.

Eventually, if you meditate consistently and train the mind to return to the now over and over again, you will start to see, feel, and sense yourself with a whole new awareness. Naturally, the more concentrated you are on the present moment, the quieter the thinking mind becomes, and the less you distract yourself with thoughts of the past or the future. You stay present to your truest reality.

By keeping your mental focus on the breath and the body, you learn to observe the flux of emotions always moving through you without reacting to them — merely witnessing them. You stop giving your emotional body the power to control your life and your mind; you also gain power over each and every moment and how you are responding to it. Eventually, you gain control of your mind and therefore your entire life. These are the benefits of mindfulness.

Of all the yoga concepts explained by the ancient gurus, I believe this is one of the easiest to understand and the most difficult to actually implement and embody. Mindfulness practices change not only the way we think, act, and feel; these practices change the neurological programming of our brains. Before you write this step off as an easy one, I would like to share with you how difficult and profound my first intensive meditation retreat was for me.

The Meditative Yogi

Ten years ago, I took my first trip to India, the motherland of yoga. I came to India in high hopes that I would find a little enlightenment or some sort of profound spiritual revelation as I journeyed around the country. The first few weeks were downright exhausting. In fact, I can confidently tell you that I was feeling nearly every emotion other than peace, calmness, or enlightenment.

The tuk-tuk drivers were a constant source of frustration. The food, although delicious, often left my body sick and weak. The pollution and the trash along the sides of the roads left me feeling filthy and disgusted. And the on-again, off-again train adventure I was on — from the northernmost part of the country to the southern tip — left me energetically depleted and emotionally exhausted.

Every time I asked someone for directions, I would receive the answer "Just go this way, madam," along with a finger point and a little head wobble. Whatever I was looking for was rarely to be found in the direction they confidently sent me. An Indian friend told me once that the phrases "no" and "I don't know" are believed to be rude in India, so out of politeness many people will offer you an answer to your question — even if it's the wrong answer. Of course, everyone in India doesn't do this, but it's something that happened frequently in my first few months of traveling through the country.

The crowds, the sicknesses, the unpredictability, and the general discomfort of India can be overwhelming for Westerners at first, especially if you are already in a bad mood. If something frustrates you here, it seems like you always attract more of it. Wandering through a country like India, so wildly different from all other countries, offers us an incredible mirror into ourselves in a vast number of ways. I believe this is why many describe their travels in India as life changing and soul growing.

I knew it would be a wild, hair-raising adventure coming to the spiritual motherland, but I didn't realize I would spend most of my first trip simply wanting to leave. How did Gandhi and Krishnamurti manage to create peace, calm, and wisdom in such a frustrating and hectic environment?

After a few months traveling around to the most vibrantly colorful temples and experiencing the most culturally diverse population (they speak a different language in each state), I decided to lock myself away from the country — without actually leaving. I signed up for my first-ever ten-day silent meditation course in the stunningly beautiful southern state of Kerala.

When my rickshaw arrived at the gates of the Dhamma Ketana Vipassana Centre, I entered one of the most gorgeous fields of towering palm trees I had ever seen. The honks and horns of India couldn't have felt further away; the place was pure peace. The idea of sitting and meditating for ten whole days seemed absolutely perfect, as the benefits of meditation were exactly what I had come to India to find but had not been able to connect with. Now here I was, about to begin a retreat to show me how to feel peaceful.

But to my surprise, that is not what initially happened. As my tuk-tuk drove away, I felt a wave of anxiety taking over my body. Standing on the front steps of the meditation center with my overflowing backpack resting heavily on my shoulders, I could feel my heart beating out of my chest and tears dripping down the curves of my cheeks. I was petrified to sit silently, cross-legged, doing absolutely nothing, for nearly twelve hours a day for the next ten days. (To be quite honest, each of these aspects scared the shit out of me.) I would not be allowed to write, read, or talk, and we would only be permitted to eat early in the morning and once again midday.

Quickly, my overwhelm turned into sheer panic. I wanted to leave, and yet I hadn't even actually begun. Once again, I felt like I had been given the wrong directions. An overwhelming voice in my head was telling me I had made a mistake by coming here. But I decided to stay because I had a deep urge to actually "meditate," whatever that meant.

At 4:30 the next morning, a loud gong startled me out of my simple little mosquito-net-covered bed, beckoning me to enter the unadorned meditation hall next door. The first thing the teacher said to us was, "Grab a cushion and sit down." So I did. Then he didn't say anything else for the next two hours, so

I sat there on my cushion … thinking. I sat there complaining to myself about what a horrid situation I had put myself into, between bouts of falling asleep and then waking up to my head whiplashing forward toward the floor.

A few hours later, to my relief, the skinny, white-haired Indian man sitting at the front of the room instructed us to focus our mind on the edge of our nostrils and the area just below the nostrils as the breath moved in and out. He told us to simply watch the nose and feel the air flowing in and the air flowing out.

Then, there were a few more hours of silence.

For the next several days, this was my task: to watch the nose. We received surprisingly few instructions these first days, but I was passionate to learn to meditate, so I diligently sat there try-ing to focus my mind on my nose. Sounds simple, right?

Over time, I started to notice that I could actually feel the minuscule hairs in my nose moving as I breathed. Hour after hour, this is what I tried to concentrate on, but it was so diffi-cult. My mind continued to drift away to anything and every-thing my mind wanted to think about.

Songs would get stuck in my head for hours at a time — usually weird, random songs that I hadn't heard for years, songs that I didn't even realize I knew every word to until I sat silently singing along to them in my head. Then my mind would drift to situations that had happened in the past, situations I had never thought of before now. I remembered random meetings with people at a bar. I would recall their names and what they were wearing, even if I had only spent five minutes of my life with them.

But mostly, I would think about the future. I would think about the moment I would walk out of this center and feared that I would feel I had wasted so much time sitting here, sing-ing, reminiscing, and daydreaming.

Each day I would wake up at 4:30 a.m. and meditate until 6:30. Then the gong would sound, allowing me to move into the dining hall for breakfast. After eating, we were given a little break to bathe and rest before returning to meditate for a long four-hour stint. These four-hour sessions were the bane of my daily existence. Sitting in that room for those hours was torturous.

To my relief, 240 minutes later, when the gong finally sounded again, everyone in the room would slowly get up and make their way to the dining hall for our last meal of the day. I didn't move slowly; I often raced there. The greatest joy of those ten days was, without a doubt, eating.

After lunch, once again I would return to the meditation hall, and, as in all the other sitting sessions in that hall, I would attempt to keep my mind focused on the breath moving in and out of my nose. I often found myself getting frustrated at my inability to successfully complete this simple task.

Sometimes during the meditation session I would start counting down the hours, minutes, and seconds until tea time, distracting myself from the present moment and fully focusing on the future. Tea time was another favorite highlight of my days during the retreat. I was always eager to leave my medita-tion cushion, and that deeply frustrated me. I would often go off on a frustration tangent for a little while before remember-ing to redirect my awareness back to my nose again.

I kept asking myself, "Why can't you simply sit here and focus on your nose, Kori? It is incredibly simple, and yet you can't manage to do it." I found myself very discouraged throughout the process — or, to be more accurate, I should say my mind was flooded with discouraging thoughts of myself.

Every evening I would intently listen to the teacher tell us stories about the struggles we were going through, which made us all laugh. Apparently, the mental roller-coaster ride I was experiencing was absolutely normal for beginning meditators, but knowing that still didn't make the process any easier or change the efficiency of my practice. Finally, to my relief, around 9 p.m. we could return to bed, our thin sleeping mattresses all wrapped up in frayed old mosquito netting.

The first three days were downright difficult. Most of the time I felt I wasn't progressing as a meditator. Halfway through day three, I started to feel more in touch with my nose than a retired ear, nose, and throat doctor. Even though my practice felt incredibly broken, I did manage to return my awareness to my nose here and there throughout each session.

It came as a rude awakening on day four when the teacher announced to the class, "Today I will teach you vipassana meditation." My mind started silently cussing the teacher out: "Excuse me, sir? Let me get this right: you are telling me that I haven't even started meditating yet? So ... what the hell have I been doing this whole time? Dear God, please let this experience just end already. I have wasted so much time. I could be seeing more of India!" I was not floating in the clouds like I imagined I would be, and that made me incredibly frustrated.

The first three days we learned a meditation technique called *anapanasati*, meaning "mindfulness of breathing" in Sanskrit; it is used to develop the mind's ability to concentrate. Our teacher told us this was the meditation style most often taught by the Buddha. We were learning to focus on one thing, and that one thing we were directed to focus on was the sensations of the nose. Unbeknownst to me at the time, this meditation technique is a prerequisite to the more advanced technique of meditation, vipassana, which we learned on day four.

Without the ability to concentrate, it is nearly impossible to become aware of what is actually happening within you. *Vipassana* means "insight" in Sanskrit. Vipassana is where you take your newly developed ability to concentrate and scan your entire body with it from head to toe. In my first moments practicing vipassana, I felt a tingling sensation coming from the hairs on the top of my scalp. As I moved my awareness down the body, I noticed sweat dripping down from my breasts to the skin of my stomach. I found intense muscle knots hardening around my hips from all of the hours I spent sitting cross-legged.

My teacher explained that by watching what was happening within the mind and body — like these sensations of tingling, dripping, and pain — and not reacting to them, we were learning how to become equanimous. *Equanimous* means remaining unaffected, neither enjoying nor disliking, staying completely unbiased and neutral toward whatever is happening. We were learning to simply observe ourselves without engaging in emotional reactivity to whatever arose.

By remaining equanimous throughout our meditation, we were training the mind to associate thoughts, sensations, and feelings, not with being pleasurable and good or unpleasant and bad, but simply with what is. The teacher explained that by developing an equanimous mind through these two meditation techniques, we were retraining the brain to stop riding the roller coaster of life, so we could just sit back and watch it in peace.

Essentially, this practice was teaching me not to habitually get anxious as the rickety cart moved up the roller-coaster track and, similarly, not to hold on with white knuckles as the cart started free-falling back down. If you meditate enough, you learn to stay balanced and nonreactive through the entire ride, which allows you to enjoy the process in its entirety. Apparently, as I was told by the teacher, when we learn to do this, life becomes a much more peaceful experience.

However, I was still fully engaged in the roller-coaster ride my mind was taking me on. By day six, despite all the valuable teachings I was receiving and gradual progress I was making, my mind got mean. I sat before the peaceful teacher with tears streaming down my cheeks, and I asked him, "Sir, I am so confused. It seems impossible to neither like the good and happy moments nor dislike the pain and things I am averse to. The pain in my hips seems only to be getting worse the more hours I sit here, and I am certain that nothing in this entire life will make me like this feeling. I want it to go away. I don't want to sit here anymore. It's not only not working, but it is really hurting me."

He responded to me in the softest and calmest of voices: "My child, why do you mention the future? Today is only day six. Tell me, how is day six going? So you are in pain? Sit and cry if you need to while meditating, but stay with what is happening right now in each moment, with each breath."

I put my head down and started to walk out of the meditation hall when he called to me so everyone could hear: "And be happy." I looked back to see his white teeth glowing through his genuine smile. Although the process was proving to be immensely challenging for me, my eighty-something-year-old Indian teacher, who appeared to never readjust his legs or check the clock to see how much time was left in the meditation session, seemed to be floating, happily. So once again, even though I wanted to leave, I stayed.

By day eight, I was absolutely fed up with it all. I wanted to eat after 11:30 a.m. I did not want to wake up at 4:30 a.m. to sit in a dark, quiet room, trying to meditate while half-asleep. I started to create stories in my head about my fellow women meditators sitting beside me, whom I had never even spoken to.

A few rows ahead of me sat a young, dreadlocked hippie girl who always wore large and baggy T-shirts. Her T-shirt would often slip off the edge of her bony shoulder, revealing her skin. This really irritated me. Despite the fact that I had spent most of my adolescence prancing around in Brazilian-style bikinis, I found it incredibly offensive and distracting for her to so carelessly show her skin. This was against the rules! I simply wouldn't stand for it, but what could I do?

Another meditator in the room was an older Muslim lady who would take a banana off the fruit tray every day during tea time, despite the fact that we were forbidden to eat at that hour. I found her daily rule-breaking habit infuriating as well. Sometimes I would sit for two hours just wondering how they could live with themselves for blatantly breaking rules the way they did.

But the worst offender that week was actually a young local woman from a nearby village whose dark hair reached down to her bum. She would sit through every four-hour meditation session completely undisturbed, like a marble statue. She obviously came here often. She was like a beautiful, enlightened female version of the Dalai Lama. As I watched her meditating, I kept thinking to myself, "How is she doing it? How is she just sitting there, never even opening her eyes for a second, completely in the zone? How is she doing this with so much peace?" I was jealous; I wanted that peace. But I couldn't have it because I was too distracted by her peace.

Then again, usually minutes later, my mind would return to singing another random Beach Boys or Frank Zappa song, or I would take unnecessary bathroom breaks, or I would day-dream for another twenty, forty, sixty minutes at a time. Truth be told, here and there, I did manage to meditate a little, too.

On day nine, I started worrying less about what the others were doing and focusing more on the sensations constantly ebbing and flowing through me. It felt as if I was slowly awak-ening to all the atoms moving within my body. This certainly seemed like some sort of a breakthrough, so in my mind I jumped for joy, sang praises to myself, and smiled so brightly you couldn't wipe the happiness off my unequanimous face. I quickly realized, with disappointment, that I was doing exactly what the teacher had told me I was to stop doing: reacting. Dang, hadn't I learned anything?

For the rest of the day, the sensations of my body be-came fluid like water. From the top of my head to the tips of my toes, I would scan my entire body with each breath. I didn't notice the excruciating pain in my hips anymore, and I started looking at the clock on the wall behind me a little less frequently.

There were still plenty of distractions, but they seemed to be appearing less. With each hour that I sat and meditated, time on my cushion seemed to flow with increasing ease. When I re-alized that I was improving at meditation, I would cheer myself on: "Go me, go me, go me. But wait … that's not equanimous."

On the final day, the teacher told us, "It takes a lifetime to perfect these teachings if you are very lucky; otherwise it may take many lifetimes. You must practice diligently, remain patient, be persistent … and be happy." And there it was again, that same huge white smile I had first seen just days before.

I spent the last days of the retreat watching the sensations flowing through me. I noticed how, when a particular thought came to my mind, it often led to an emotion, and those feelings morphed into some sort of reaction. When I focused more intently on the inhale and exhale that were always happening, minimizing the distractions of my thinking mind, I started to notice a calm peacefulness inside me. I could feel the impermanence of everything in life; everything was constantly changing, which made it easier not to react to it. Aha!

I loved the calm and peaceful feeling, but I knew I couldn't grasp onto this either, for it too was destined to pass away. For the first time in ten days, I realized that when I focused my mind on the reality of now — whatever the now might look like — and did not react, everything always seemed to be okay! It dawned on me that this was actually the point of all of this time sitting: not to eliminate thoughts, feelings, and sensations, but to react to them less. That is what meditation was teaching me.

On the tenth day, when I heard the last 4:30 a.m. gong blasts of the retreat, I got out of bed and walked to the meditation hall more slowly than ever. Suddenly, I wasn't in a hurry anymore. Two hours later, I didn't rush to the dining hall for breakfast, either.

As I walked to breakfast, finally moving slowly and thoughtfully, my eyes caught a glimpse of the most delicate bundle of purple flowers growing just beside the pathway. I realized that in my usual rush to eat breakfast, craving food and distracted by the obsessions of my thinking mind, I had carelessly failed to notice the flowers blooming along my short daily walk. The flowers were morning glories, blooming only in the dawn chill before closing into hibernation for the rest of the day.

These flowers had opened every single morning of the retreat, and yet I had not been able to see or appreciate them until now, ten full days of meditation later. I thought to myself, "Has it really taken me ten days of silent stillness to slow my mind enough to stop and notice the flowers?" Thankfully, here I was seeing the benefits of ten days of mindfulness practice with my own eyes.

As I packed my backpack to leave, I did it with a mindful concentration on each shirt I folded. As I sipped on my last cup of chai, I watched the dew dissipate from the morning grass and listened to the song of the birds as they playfully bounced from tree to tree. These ten days of meditating taught me to live more mindfully in the present moment, to observe everything in the now. With my newfound skill, I could finally stop and smell, not just those sweet little morning glories, but the flowers of my soul that were just begging me to notice them.

Finally, it was time to leave. With my backpack on I walked out to the road and waved down a small pickup truck. I asked the driver if he would drop me at the local train station. He said yes, of course. I suddenly realized that perhaps this tendency for Indians to say yes was actually an effect of their more open mindset, one where anything and everything is possible.

As I jumped in the back bed of the pickup truck and clung to the metal rack just above the cab, I felt like a high school homecoming queen standing tall and proud, waving to the children who ran out of their mud farm shacks to get a closer look at me. My hair blew wildly in the wind as we sped down the small rural roads. The full moon was still visible in the midmorning sky. I noticed in that moment how peaceful I felt now that I was living in the present, not in a hurry or anxious to get to the train station, but seeing everything as it passed by. For the first time on my trip in India, I could actually appreciate what was rather than what I expected it to be.

Now I felt that I was ready for India. I too started to adopt the mindset that I could get anywhere from any direction. I started to expand my limiting beliefs to see that everything is possible. I began to understand the power of surrender and floating, which were so necessary for peacefully traveling through India. Luckily, the ten-day meditation retreat gave me just that.

Meditation

As the story of my first meditation retreat clearly shows, starting a meditation practice is hard, and I have discovered it is equally challenging to stay consistent with it day in and day out. But when I regularly meditate, I have found it to be one of the most effective life-changing practices the yogis offered us for connecting with the peaceful, calm, inner golden soul of myself.

When you meditate, you are not simply learning to quiet the mind; more importantly, you are learning to not react to the mind so you can stay calm and collected in the present. While it can feel like a waste of time in the beginning, every little bit of meditation you do retrains your mind to stay detached from the ebbs and flows of thoughts and emotions moving within, teaching you to have a single-pointed focus on what's happening in the now.

In the world we live in, we have a natural tendency to hurry ourselves up and focus on reaching our goals, rather than resting in the present moment and feeling what is happening within us. At my first meditation retreat, I was focused on my own goals and expectations rather than on the flowers I walked past every day.

Similarly, it was the same future focus on what I expected to find during my trip to India that actually made me hate it at first.

Mindfulness has taught me to see everything differently. Mindfulness is about simply realizing how you feel right here, right now, and not reacting to it. That's it. Meditation is the practice the yogis offered us to do just that. It is the principal practice offered by the Buddha as well.

Just as we create space in the physical layer for intuitive messages to seep to the surface of our consciousness, mindfulness creates space in the mental layer for them to do the same. When spaciousness meets mindfulness, you are well on your way to hearing and feeling your intuitive messages. With an open and expansive physical body and a calm, concentrated mind, you become aware of how you are feeling as it is happening, and that is just perfect if you want to connect with the world of your inner soul.

Knowing what you want in your life and what you would like to see happen in the future is important — don't get me wrong — but racing to get there will make the journey absolutely miserable for you. In fact, without mindfulness, it's hard to feel the intuitive messages rising up from within you. Similarly, without mindfulness, manifestation is damn near impossible.

You have to move into the body for as many present moments as you possibly can in order to hear those messages loud and clear. Then you must remain focused on the here and now to be able to see all the opportunities the universe is constantly sending you to make those dreams your reality. And you will.

Humans are a lot like oysters in the way we build a thick shell around us. Ours is made of distraction and mental busyness. It's a form of protection, a way to keep unwanted feelings out, but it also locks our mind into the pain we are feeling, and all of our actions in turn become reactions to that pain. These protective layers — the busyness, the distraction, and the monkey mind — disconnect us from our natural state of happiness, calm, and presence, which is always there inside you, vibrating out from your soul. The academic researcher and bestselling author Brené Brown, who studies shame and vulnerability, explains that "'crazy-busy' is a great armor, it's a great way for numbing. What a lot of us do is that we stay so busy, and so out in front of our life, that the truth of how we're feeling and what we really need can't catch up with us."

Unlike oysters, we don't need a shell. Meditation helps us break it down, leaving us strong and accepting of our vulnerability to be who our soul wants us to be. One of the greatest benefits I have received from my meditation practice is that I have learned to perceive the world around me for what it actually is, not what I project it to be or want it to be. Meditation allows us to start seeing the world from the pearl at your center, rather than blocking that reality with the shell on the outside. This is why many refer to meditation as "the art of living."

Breath

Breath is a natural tool for staying in the present moment. Mindful breathing practices, otherwise known as meditations, are techniques offered by Buddhists and yogis alike for retraining the mind to live in the present moment. Watching and playing with the breath is the yoga step called *pranayama*, meaning "breath awareness" in Sanskrit.

Focusing on the breath is the simplest form of meditation. In following the in and out of the breath, the up and down of the chest, the soft lifting and falling of the shoulders, you learn that everything is constantly changing. Everything has changed. Everything will change. Simply by watching the breath, you learn to be at peace with change.

When it comes to maintaining a healthy mind, conscious breathing is the key. Breathing alone helps you learn to control your reactions and remain calm. Breathing has a major effect on other parts of the body as well, and it can contribute to your overall health and happiness. When your mind is overcome with anger, your breath is the first element in your body to physically react. Whether you are worried, scared, heartbroken, or happy, the breath reacts to these feelings. By learning to be mindful of what is happening to your breath, you become more aware of how you are feeling in each moment.

Breathing meditations connect us not only to ourselves but also to our surroundings. As you inhale, the chemistry of the air molecules and the energetic charge of the air come into the body and are immediately assessed by the hypothalamus in the brain. The brain translates this "air quality report" to the rest of the body via a million blood vessels. This is how the breath helps us harmonize with the environment.

As you breathe in, you take the unseen energy floating all around you and pull it inside your body. You absorb what you need and release what you don't. Your breath acts as a bridge linking the energy from inside the body to the outside, from the soul to the universe.

When mountaineers climb to the tallest mountain peaks in the world, they stop several times along the way so their body can acclimate to the increasing altitude. These acclimatization days allow the body to equalize with the new environment. When mountaineers are nearly to the summit of Mount Everest, for example, the body can sense the thinness of the air, and the lungs adjust to breathe more slowly. Acclimatizing requires transformation of the breath.

Similarly, the body must evolve as the world around us changes. Anatomically, as the air from outside your body moves inside through your nostrils, the breath nurtures and sustains every single cell of your physical body, which nurtures your mental and therefore your spiritual body. Whether you are 20,000 feet up in the air or in a life-threatening situation or lying comfortably on your bed, the breath communicates to the body what needs to happen to keep you alive.

As the body translates what is happening around you, your gut may react by sending you a sensation of butterflies; your heart may skip a beat. The more deeply you learn to feel, the better you can read the body and the messages moving throughout it. This is how you become fluent in the language of your intuition.

As you pay attention to your inhalations and exhalations, lifelong habits of the mind change, new neural pathways develop in the brain, and you start seeing things from a very different perspective. Scientific research has proven that breathing practices physically alter the prefrontal cortex, which is involved in focus, planning, and impulse control. Controlled breathing raises your levels of dopamine, making you happier. Breathing practices can treat depression, anxiety, anger issues, and attention deficiencies, among many other struggles. Breath work can heal the mind as well as retrain it.

Professional athletes use these yogic breathing techniques before championship games in order to improve their performance. Businesspeople and life coaches like Tony Robbins credit breathing practices with guiding their own business growth and life decisions. One of my favorite examples of the power of the breath is Wim Hof, known as "the Iceman." Hof is an extreme athlete who preaches breathing practices and meditation as part of his Wim Hof Method.

Hof set Guinness World Records for swimming under ice and still holds the record for a barefoot half marathon on ice and snow. He also set the world record for the longest time in direct, full-body contact with ice and has climbed to an altitude of 7,200 meters on Mount Everest wearing nothing but shorts and shoes. In February 2009, Hof reached the top of Mount Kilimanjaro, and then in September, he ran a full marathon in the Namib Desert without water. Breathing practices and meditation are not just for the spiritual seekers anymore; they are helpful for anyone on a mission to become or create anything in their lives.

Yoga masters such as Yajnavalkya, Vyasa, Shankaracharya, and Patanjali, as well as Vedic and tantric scriptures, recognize breath work as one of the greatest tools for connecting to your soul. In Hebrew, Greek, Sanskrit, Mayan, Hawaiian, and Latin, *spirit* and *breath* are strikingly similar words in sound and in meaning. Across cultures, breath represents the movement of spirit within the human body. It's a sign the body is alive and working.

Personally, I like to think of my breathing as a constant prayer. Inhalations are the part of the universe that I take into myself, and exhalations are what I put out to the universe. Your breath has been with you since the day you were born and will constantly flow through you until the day you die. If anything is sacred, it is breath. If there is a connection to God, I believe the breath must be it.

Your breath takes your deepest heartfelt desires and asks the universe to help you manifest them. I believe your prayers gain power through mindfulness and conscious breathing, which are the tools you learn through practicing pranayama techniques. The more mindful of your breath you become, the more power the prayers you inhale and exhale will be.

4

The Meditations

If you begin to understand what you are without trying to change it,
then what you are undergoes a transformation.

— JIDDU KRISHNAMURTI

As my seasonal work in Alaska was coming to an end one summer, I felt a strong urge to go to Africa. A travel partner and I bought one-way tickets to Nairobi, Kenya, where we would begin an arduous journey through the southeast region of the continent. I can't remember what exactly motivated this particular trip, but I am confident the dream arose as all dreams do, to teach me something deep and soulful. The three months I spent traveling across Africa taught me a lot about the power of my meditation practice. Through this journey, I learned to stay calm in the presence of difficulties and to appreciate the moments of magic that were always destined to appear thereafter.

We chose not to take a tour or join one of the overland buses traveling through the country, like most young travelers do; we wanted to see Africa from the locals' perspective. To get an honest and real look at the parts of the continent we would travel through, we took public transportation as much as possible. In my twenties, I prided myself on not being a tourist. I preferred calling myself a traveler, less focused on the sites I wanted to check off my list and more interested in being open to whatever the journey showed me. I wanted to travel through the continent in as unprivileged a way as a privileged young woman could. As uncomfortable as this trip might prove to be, I wanted to step away from my industrialized country convenience and really experience something wildly different.

We didn't have fixed plans regarding where we would go or how long it would take us to get there, but I knew I would like to end this trip in Cape Town, South Africa, and fly home from there. Logistically, this would be the best place from which to get a flight home. It would also offer me the posh hotel room and chilled glass of wine I felt I would deserve when I finally made it to the finish line of such a grand adventure.

Upon arrival in Nairobi, I already knew I was well out of my comfort zone. As we drove from the airport to our dilapidated hotel room, my eyes were glued to the dry, dusty landscapes we passed through and the people sitting alongside the road simply trying to survive. Skinny children walked beside the rusty old Toyota Corolla taxi we were in, banging on the window to get our attention, selling everything from hangers to cellphone chargers. My taxi driver — whom I could clearly tell was sick by the way his skin sunk into his deep and dark eye sockets — told us stories of how hard life was for him, stories of constant misfortunes. From our first moments on the continent, the message was clear: life indeed was full of suffering.

Many of the people we met along the way had incredibly challenging lives, amplified by colonization and class inequalities. When it came to struggles, I realized I had very few.

We took the bus from Kenya to Tanzania before jumping on a train headed south to Zambia. Everything seemed to be going swimmingly, until we were stopped quite literally on our train tracks on the southern border of Tanzania. We were surprised to hear that all public transportation bound south toward Zambia was unavailable, as the government had reallocated most of the buses, trains, and ferryboats to bring fleeing Congolese refugees away from their war-torn country and into Tanzania.

Of course, I was grateful that the Tanzanian government was helping the displaced and struggling Congolese refugees, but as a traveler I found myself stuck at the end of a dead end road. Along this trip my travel partner and I found ourselves running into one roadblock after another. After contemplating our choices and talking to many locals about where to go next, we ended up sharing a twelve-seater minivan taxi with twenty-four other passengers crammed inside. It was a long, hot, and uncomfortable car ride through the country.

On the way, we saw thousands of simple wooden caskets for sale along the roadside. The caskets were much too small for an average adult; they were for children. We drove past a fatal vehicle accident, bodies lying limp and lifeless on the grass beside the wreckage. I will never forget what I saw on that drive through Zambia. The reality of the suffering surrounding us was undeniable.

Exhausted and emotionally overwhelmed upon arrival in the capital city, we made it to our simple hostel beds just as sweat began pouring out of my body. My temperature quickly fluctuated between freezing cold and burning hot. Now it seemed I had contracted malaria and was fully engrossed in my own sufferings.

As I rolled from side to side in agony on the hard mattress, all I wanted to do was to return to the comfort of the past, my home back in America. Initially I had wanted to take this trip to see what life was like in East Africa, but when the discomfort arose, my impulse was to push it all away.

A few days later, we were once again ready to continue on; we were diligent about reaching the finish line no matter how challenging the journey to get there proved to be. I must admit, while this expedition was by far the toughest I had ever experienced as a modern-day explorer — or at least that is what I liked to call myself — there was always a magical reward that came after each of the hardships we encountered. That is exactly what the journey of meditation is like also: tough but rewarding. It requires diligence and determination. It isn't always easy, but it is a powerful tool for dealing with the struggles that are so intrinsically a part of human existence for all of us.

While most of the people surrounding me were dealing with horrific tragedies, such as hunger, war, poverty, and disease, my struggles lived in the workings of my mind: depression and anxiety. As minor as my difficulties might have seemed in comparison, through the miles of that long trip, I learned a lot about being with my hardships rather than constantly pushing them away or trying to get away from them. I learned to be with what was, even if it wasn't what I wanted.

Along the 5,000-mile journey, we stopped and swam in rock pools above the impressive Victoria Falls, a magical place where a thick 800-meter blanket of water tumbles over a wide wall of earth, seemingly stretching as far as the eye can see. In Namibia, we hiked up the largest sand dunes in the world and looked out over expansive desert lands containing more skeletons than living animals. In South Africa, we camped in countless national parklands, enjoying a glass of chilled wine at the end of the day and falling asleep to the cackling of wild hyenas and the loud foot poundings of zebras running in the distance. The most memorable moments of the trip for me were the vibrant drum and dance parties celebrating weddings and the birth of children in the smallest of towns with names I cannot remember.

In one small village in Zambia, we were invited to the local orphanage, where nearly fifty children ran up to us and followed us around for the day. Just before we left, a few of the older children asked us to dance with them. We agreed, and immediately one of the nuns pulled a few rustic hand drums from the corner of the room. A beautiful four-year-old girl adorned in a sweet white dress caught my eye as she shyly walked to the center of the room. She started to move her hips from side to side as quickly as her skinny ten-year-old brother could bang the drum. They laughed, smiled, danced, and drummed with immense excitement. They were having so much fun. When one of the little boys grabbed my hand and pulled me into the dance circle, I excitedly joined in.

The journey, in Africa as well as in meditation, is not to focus on the suffering; it is to make sure the suffering isn't keeping you from dancing when the opportunities arise. Many of us want to learn to meditate to eliminate our struggles, but meditation doesn't get rid of our struggles. It teaches us to be with ourselves and whatever arises — the good, the bad, the uncomfortable — and simply observe these moments as they pass.

I have traveled to more than fifty countries, and this trip was the most challenging as well as the most rewarding journey

I have ever taken. I can now tell you that the success of the undertaking came about because I learned to let the struggles happen without freaking out and to keep moving whenever the timing felt right. Looking back on it now, I see that this was possible only because of the diligence, patience, and persistence I learned through meditation those years past in India.

My travel partner, who was also an avid meditator, and I were resilient when it came to focusing on the now and moving forward from that place. Perhaps my soul sent me on this journey to show me how to accept not only the suffering in myself but the suffering of the entire world as a natural element of our humanness — to learn to be at peace with it.

The Buddha's first noble truth is "Life is suffering." His life purpose thereafter was to teach meditation as a tool for dealing with the inevitable suffering. I reminded myself of this many times during my adventure through Africa. There will be hardships; keep meditating.

Over the course of our adventure, we focused on the baby steps we needed to take each day, not on the overwhelming uncertainties that lay ahead of us. Our mindful presence made it possible to keep going. We were diligent about getting on the next train, bus, or shared taxi that would continue bringing us closer to Cape Town. When we practice meditation with the same diligence, we come to the peaceful place we so deeply desire.

Three months later and thirty pounds lighter, we finally did arrive in the beautiful coastal city of Cape Town. It felt like a miracle in many ways. You can be sure that I had plenty of chilled glasses of wine at trendy, posh seaside restaurants. We watched the golden sunset colors illuminating the iconic Table Mountain in the evenings and walked in the cold, raw air along the Atlantic Ocean in the mornings. The feelings that came over me at the end of the trip reminded me of that day when I left my first meditation retreat. I had the same satisfied feeling of accomplishment and momentary bliss as I had holding on to the back of the truck in India.

In Africa, I learned how to deal with suffering in an honest and peaceful way. Meditation in many ways feels like a hero's journey. It is so much easier to stick to your habitual routines and not make the time or commitment to meditate, but I want to assure you that life will become so much calmer when you do. You learn to be with your suffering and still dance.

Oftentimes the journey, especially in the beginning, feels too difficult, and the benefits seem distant and hard to imagine. I believe new meditators have the misconception that they will have fewer thoughts or struggles when they learn how to meditate, which isn't true. In fact, initially, it feels like you have more thoughts, because suddenly you can see them all. Meditation simply teaches us not to react to them. In this way meditation indirectly brings more happiness into our lives, because we learn to get ourselves unstuck from the pain and suffering as they arise.

Meditation offers a sort of self-created superpower for staying calm and becoming less reactionary when the going gets rough. To do the unthinkable, you must retrain the way you think.

During my first meditation retreat in India, the head teacher, S. N. Goenka, would tell us, "You must work patiently, persistently, and continuously. Continuity of practice is the secret of success." He was right. There is only one way to practice meditation: patiently, persistently, and continuously. Similarly, that was exactly how I would get through Africa.

I repeated this quote many times throughout my African journey. I also keep this quote tacked to my wall at home. If you practice meditation patiently, persistently, and continuously, there truly are no limits to what you can accomplish and the benefits you can receive. So practice as if your life depends on it, because your soul life actually does!

In this chapter, I offer you a collection of meditation styles and practices to choose from. As we continue our exploration into the final four stages of the yoga system in the upcoming chapters, many of the later practices will build on the mindfulness you will gain by making the practices in this chapter nonnegotiable.

The Buddha taught that mindfulness increases two qualities: *shamatha* (calm) and *vipassana* (insight and intuition). Looking back at my travels through Africa, I can see how my meditation practice helped me stay calm when both logistics and my body seemed to be failing me. My meditation practice also taught me how to think outside the box and to be creative in figuring out how we could continue moving forward when it seemed like we had arrived at yet another dead end.

As you train your mind to live in the present moment, you gradually change the way your mind has habitually functioned, making it easier to do pretty much anything — from calming anger and anxieties to traveling overland for thousands of miles just because your heart is fully set on doing it. No matter what it is you want, meditation is going to be the vehicle to get you there.

How Meditation Works

When you understand how something works, you are more likely to use it. To better understand mindful meditation, imagine that your mind is an attic filled with boxes stuffed with memories, experiences, and feelings. To truly comprehend the dimensions of the attic, you must clear out the boxes or at least organize and move things around a little bit. Meditation is the light bulb allowing you to see what is in the attic. You will be amazed at what you have been storing in there.

The mind is made up of three different components: awareness or consciousness (the light bulb); the thinking mind (the attic); and the memories and feelings (the clutter of boxes in the attic). When you meditate, your heightened awareness may bring to light the voices cluttering your mind and never-before-felt sensations on the skin of your body. Meditating isn't always going to feel peaceful and calming; you may experience anger, sadness, frustration, jealousy, or guilt. Traumatic events or distant memories may resurface. You may, for example, have a resurgence of memories of someone who is no longer with you, and that may bring you both joy and sadness.

As you move through waves of emotions, seeing all the memories that live within your mind, you transition into your natural state of being, open and expansive. You clean the attic. In the same way that we discussed creating space in your body earlier, you develop mindfulness by creating space in the mind.

People often tell me that they do not have the time to meditate. But even if you're a busy person, you can find some way to bring mindfulness into every waking hour of your life. You don't have to breathe like the quintessential cross-legged yogi on a cushion in order to meditate; you can bring awareness to your breath any time of the day, while doing anything.

When you first begin meditating, I suggest committing to a certain amount of time to familiarize yourself with the practice and ensure you create a healthy habit. Set a timer, even if it's just for five minutes in the beginning, and then add a minute each day. It's best if you can work up to trying the different practices below for at least fifteen minutes each. If something feels good to you, keep it in mind for your own mindful rituals. This is how you find what works best for you: by feeling your way to the practices that resonate with you most.

Just within the three types of breathing techniques I describe here, there are hundreds of variations to play with. What follows are the foundational practices, but if you know other breathing practices that work for you, by all means consider using those when creating your rituals.

Meditation Posture: *Padmasana*

When you meditate, it's preferable to sit up rather than lie down because it keeps the mind more alert; you'll be less inclined to fall asleep. Therefore, start in a seated position that feels comfortable and steady. Place cushions beneath your hips or your knees if this helps, or sit in a chair or even on the edge of your bed or couch if that feels better for you. When you take a similar posture every time you meditate, your muscle memory will help you transition more easily into a meditative state each time.

The classic yogi meditation posture is called Padmasana, or Lotus position. This is often how the Buddha is depicted in temples and paintings. Simply sit on the floor with your legs crossed, either fully crossed in the Lotus position or loosely crossed, whichever is most comfortable for you. From this position, begin lifting your posture from the crown of the head, growing a tall, long spine. Allow the tailbone to ground itself in the opposite direction of your head while you inhale and lengthen through the spine. Soon, you will be able to exhale, soften, and relax into this position without trying.

Tuck your chin toward your chest just a little, giving your spine more freedom. Lightly press the tip of the tongue against the roof of your mouth just behind your upper row of teeth. Roll your shoulders back and down, finding a neutral posture. Now, mentally scan through the body, and if you notice tension, make subtle movements to help you feel more comfortable. Place your hands in your lap with your left hand on top, palm facing upward.

While this is the most common meditation pose, you can meditate in any position. If you find this posture difficult, simply sit in a chair or on the couch with a straight spine to keep you alert. The most important thing is to make sure that you are comfortable and the body feels soft. Ultimately, you are training yourself to meditate in all positions, while walking, talking, and moving about your life, so feel free to experiment with different postures and then stick with the one that feels the most steady and comfortable to you.

The Mindfulness Practices

Before you move on to the meditations in this chapter, keep in mind that this book is not intended to read like many others; it is not meant to be a speedy page-turner. This book is meant to be a resource. I encourage you to spend time practicing each meditation. Take breaks between each chapter to sit with the concepts and think about how you can integrate them into your life.

If you are inspired and ready to run forward on your spiritual path, which I hope you are, then breeze through the pages and create your rituals immediately, but please do come back to the practices below and refresh your rituals or create new ones in the future. This will guarantee that your yoga practices still resonate strongly with you wherever you are in each present moment.

The Meditative Natural Breathing Practices

The first breathing technique I will teach you is meditative natural breathing, the basic introduction to meditation. Simply by watching your breath as it moves in and out of the nose, you are training your mind to focus. Here are two versions of the practice.

The Mindfulness of Breathing Practice

The first meditation I ever learned is called *anapanasati*, or "mindfulness of breathing." This meditation was originally taught by the Buddha himself and has since been adopted by Tibetan, Zen, Tiantai, Theravada, and Western meditation schools. Nearly every style of meditation around the world begins with this practice, which is based on focusing your concentration on the sensations around the nostrils.

In a comfortable meditation position (whatever that looks like for you), close your eyes and bring your awareness to the tip of your nose. Feel the breath move in and out of the body without changing your breathing in any way.

Let the breath flow in its own natural rhythm, and just observe it.

As the mind wanders, which it will, compassionately and patiently refocus your awareness back on the nostrils and the upper lip. When the mind drifts off to thoughts, this does not mean that you have failed or had a "bad" session. Distractions are opportunities for retraining the mind to become more mindful.

The Zen Breath Counting Practice

In the Zen Buddhist tradition, the Zen breath counting meditation practice is taught to first-time meditators as a technique for increasing your ability to concentrate by giving you a subtle action to focus on: in this case, counting the breath.

Begin by taking a deep breath in, silently say, "One," and then exhale, silently saying, "One" again. Slowly and softly inhale, mentally say, "Two," and then exhale, mentally saying, "Two." Continue breathing like this, counting each breath until you reach ten. Then work your way backward down to one. When you lose track of what number you last said, which you inevitably will, simply begin again at one.

Many of us lose our focus; even lifelong monks have some days when they are more unfocused than others. Try not to become tense or frustrated as this happens; calmly continue counting as the breath naturally moves in and out. If you are doing the practice, you are developing mindfulness, which means you are learning to focus and live in the present moment.

If you confidently count up to ten and back a few times in a row, then make it a little more challenging and increase your counting to twenty. Buddhist masters have claimed that when you can consciously breathe up to one hundred and back down to one again, you will have developed such inner power that you'll be able to achieve anything in life you set your mind to. In other words, you are developing your ability to create your own reality.

Zen breath counting is one of the best practices for

beginners because you can actually watch your mind growing more mindful as your ability to increase the count improves. At first, you may be able to stay focused on your breath only up to the count of four, but a few days later you may find yourself staying focused up to the count of twenty or thirty. Every day is different, every moment is different, and the number you can count to on any given day will differ.

Rather than look at this practice as something you are improving, try to look at it as an exploration of where your ability to concentrate is in this exact moment, without any judgments or labels.

The Body-Scanning Practice

Once you are familiar with the natural breathing meditations above, then you can slowly begin guiding your newfound mindful concentration through your entire body. The body-scanning meditation practice below works by bringing mindfulness into each part of the body with your inhale and exhale. The more mindfully you move your awareness through the body, the more your body will soften and release.

Mindfulness naturally promotes relaxation. In this practice, you will not only be learning to maintain mindfulness but also creating relaxation in the body.

Instead of trying to do the practice while reading the instructions, you can record the guided meditation on your phone and then listen to it.

A Guided Body-Scanning Meditation

This practice can be performed while lying down, sitting, or in any relaxing position with your eyes closed. Take a few breaths in silence before you begin body scanning. Then, while inhaling, visualize your body as it fills up with a fresh supply of oxygen. Exhale and silently say to yourself, "And relax."

Now, begin the meditation by bringing your awareness to the crown of your head. Inhale and exhale mindfully into your forehead, focusing your attention on that part of the body. Then do the same with your eyes, eye sockets, cheekbones, ears, mouth, and jaw, using the inhale and exhale to move your attention to each part in turn. With each inhale, feel the sensations present in your entire face, and as you exhale without trying, observe the muscles in your face relax.

You can take as many breaths into each body part as you choose to. You may wish to stay in some areas a little longer, or, conversely, you might take only one breath into each body part. Let your intuition guide the length of time you spend in each area.

Take a few extra breaths into the jaw, an area of the body that tends to hold tension. Next, begin breathing into your neck and throat. Move the focus of your breathing into your shoulders, upper chest, upper arms, elbows, lower arms, hands, palms, and fingertips. Inhale deeply through your nose and feel the exhalation pushing out, finally releasing through the tips of your fingers.

Now, bring your attention to your stomach. If it's tense or tight, let it soften and move with ease as you bring air in and let the breath flow out. If you feel a strong sensation, simply take note of it. Try not to overanalyze or label the sensation you are feeling as "good" or "bad." Just continue inhaling and exhaling and moving your conscious awareness throughout the body, observing it in its entirety, full of different sensations in different areas.

Breathe into the backside of the body. If there are places where you cannot feel any sensations — voids in your awareness — you can take a few extra breaths into these areas to bring more mindfulness and openness to them. Then continue scanning. Move your breath into the entire pelvic girdle and down into the upper legs, knees, and calves. Inhale through the nose, moving the breath through the body and out through the bottoms of the feet and the toes.

Finally, take a deep, full breath in and bring your awareness to all the cells of your body, moving your attention from the toes back up to the crown of the head. Begin with ten cycles of scanning this way or, if you prefer, mindfully move through the body for a set amount of time. On your second round, continue scanning from the crown of your head to the tips of your toes, moving your awareness through each part along the way. Sweep your breath up and down as quickly or as slowly as you feel comfortable, scanning for tension and noting your own sensations. Try not to attach any like or dislike to any of the sensations that appear along the way.

Continue in this way, stopping and tuning in to each part as you move your focus down through the body, inhaling and exhaling fully in the present moment. Rather than trying to intentionally relax the body, concentrate more on staying mindful of each area of the body, simply noticing any sensations that are present. Without reacting to them, you will find that the sensations move on their own, naturally arising and then passing away.

This is how you will begin to move through your daily life with a mindful, peaceful awareness. Naturally, relaxation will follow.

The Altered Breath Practices

Altered breathing awareness is a meditation style that changes the breath and in turn creates subtle changes within the body. If your mind tends to be scattered and easily distracted, you will find it easier to remain engaged in your meditation practice when the mind is doing something, such as extending your exhale for a specific count or alternating which nostril you breathe through.

As your mindfulness develops, you will start to see the strong connection between your mind and your physical body. For example, when you feel anxious, oftentimes your heart reacts by beating a little faster, and your hands may feel shakier. When you are depressed, you may feel lethargic and lack energy.

You may notice that when you get stressed, your diaphragm locks and tightens, limiting the depth of your breath. When your breath becomes shallow, your body can't take in oxygen, which means that blood doesn't reach your digestive organs. When this happens, your body lacks the ability to fight off illness and disease. This is why stress is so harmful to us and also why breathing through it is so deeply healing.

Seventy-five percent of the population in the Western world is affected by chronic stress. Stress impacts the way you feel, the way you think, and the way your body functions. The only way to notice the stress you are experiencing in your body is by sitting with your breath in the present moment and observing it. The natural breathing practices in this chapter help you become aware of what is happening.

As your meditation practices develop and you become more intimate with your own body, you can use altered breathing practices to help you transform particular energies. As long as you are not attached to a specific outcome and, instead, are using the altered breathing as a way to explore the connections between breath and body, you are developing your mindfulness.

The concept of moving and guiding energy is the basis behind the Eastern holistic practices of Reiki, tai chi, qigong, acupuncture, acupressure, and of course many types of yoga, especially yin yoga and chakra meditations. The more you learn about yourself through your natural breathing practices, the easier it will become for you to use the breath to create change within the body. The altered breathing practices can help you heal.

In our modern world full of hustle, we cannot avoid stress in our lives, but we can develop and practice ways to respond to it. Making a habit of conscious breathing is the key to reversing daily stress. Altered breathing techniques are effective for pain management and for minimizing the suffering in your life. In hospitals throughout the world, doctors and nurses teach specific breathing techniques to laboring mothers delivering children, to patients having intense anxiety attacks, and as a therapy for pain management.

Dr. Robert C. Fulford was an allopathic doctor who experimented with altering breathing techniques as a treatment for chronic ear infections and other lymph-related issues in children. Dr. Fulford found that by guiding children to breathe in certain ways, the body would actually remove bacteria (similar to the effects of an antibiotic). He found he could manipulate the lymphatic system to cure children's ear infections without ever prescribing them pharmaceuticals, but by teaching them how to breathe in a new way. Dr. Fulford used altered breathing practices in his own life, too, and went on to live to the ripe old age of ninety-one.

The body is one big, interconnected system. By altering the natural breath to make it deeper, slower, and longer — by lengthening, holding, or stimulating it — you can bring your body into balance. The relationship between the mind and the breath is intimate. When you are scared, your breath speeds up; when you feel grief, you may find it difficult to take a full breath. When the mind is anxious, your breath becomes erratic and short. Contrarily, when you are happy, you may take a long, deep sigh of relief.

Your success in using the altered breath to heal lies in your ability to mindfully tune in. First, acknowledge what is happening and how you are feeling, and then you can create an altered breathing practice for balancing and harmonizing the body. When you feel heavy (which means there is stagnation and inflammation in the body), practice detoxifying and energy-moving stimulation breathing. If you are a nonstop overdoer or have anxiety, practice calming breathing. For all else, practice balancing breathing or some of the meditative breathing techniques I've already described above.

The longest-living animals on Earth are serpents, elephants, and tortoises, and they also take the slowest and longest breaths. Slow, deep, extended breaths are healing. Whether you are healing the physical body, the mind, or the heart, breath is a powerful tool.

Ultimately, the healthier and more open you feel in your mind, the more ease and freedom you create for subconscious messages to rise to the surface of your awareness. These intuitive messages will always guide you on a journey to feel healthier and happier, so use them as they appear. Once again, you are not reacting to what you are feeling, but simply changing the breath as you see fit while keeping that equanimous attitude we talked about toward whatever you find along the way.

Here are a few altered breathing practices to explore.

Calming

EXTENDED EXHALE BREATHING PRACTICE

Take a deep breath in. On your next exhale, count how many seconds you can comfortably and fully exhale. Then, inhale while counting up to half of that number. For example, if you exhale to the count of eight, let your inhale count be four. Then, exhale for the count of eight. Repeat.

Take ten breaths like this.

BHRAMARI BREATHING

Take a deep inhale, then exhale with closed lips while making a buzzing sound like a bumblebee. Feel the hum vibrating through your entire body and recalibrating it. This bumblebee breathing technique is great for calming your body and mind and a wonderful practice to use before sleep.

Take ten breaths like this.

Stimulating

KAPALBHATI BREATHING

Take a deep breath in. Exhale completely with as many quick, sharp blasts out as you can, until the lungs feel empty. It is helpful to squeeze the anus each time you push air out. Then take another long, deep inhale and repeat the short blasts of exhale while pushing the air out with your diaphragm.

Begin by practicing ten breaths like this. At first you may

feel lightheaded, dizzy, or nauseous, so take breaks as needed to return to the natural meditative breath, then try again whenever you are ready. You can slowly build up to more breaths over time.

Please note that many yoga texts advise against practicing this breathing technique if you are pregnant or menstruating.

Balancing

ALTERNATE NOSTRIL BREATHING

Bring your right hand toward your face. Bend your pointer and middle fingers down into the palm. Press the tip of your thumb against the right nostril. Place your ring finger on the left cheek, gently pulling the cheek away from the nose to open the left nostril a little more. Inhale through the left nostril to the count of four. Then, with your thumb still holding the right nostril, use your ring finger to close the left nostril. With both nostrils closed, hold the breath for the same count of four. Then release your thumb and exhale through the right nostril for the same count of four. Inhale again through the right nostril, close both nostrils, and hold the breath again for four counts. Now, release the left nostril and exhale through it to finish one complete round of alternate nostril breathing.

Repeat this cycle at least ten times, but feel free to stay with the practice longer also. This meditation is helpful for balancing the right and left hemispheres of the brain, a form of whole brain integration.

The Unorthodox Breathing Practices

Unorthodox breathing practices are my own little practices for bringing more conscious breaths into my day no matter where I am. First, you must let go of the quintessential image of a meditation practice only happening while you are sitting cross-legged in the same place at the same time for every session. The truth is that you are always breathing, which means you can become a mindful breather anywhere and everywhere. When you sing, chant, exercise, and laugh, you are actually altering the natural rhythm of the breath with longer exhales, calming the body and mind. I like to turn these activities into conscious breathing practices by simply focusing on my breath while doing them.

You may choose to practice while in the shower, cooking dinner, or walking the dog. Like anything, if you make it fun and exciting, you will remember to practice more often.

Mantra Breathing

A mantra creates a rhythmic pattern with the breath. Mantras are syllables infused with a purpose, either in your own mother tongue or something exotic. The difference between mantra chanting and singing a song is that mantras have an intention — you focus on the sounds you are creating — whereas singing can be more unconscious. Sometimes you sing the words of a song that you aren't thinking about.

Mantras are meditative because they offer us something to focus on besides the subtle flow of our breath. Whether you choose to use an incredibly long Gregorian chant or a short and sweet yoga mantra (such as "Om"), by focusing on the breath as you chant, you turn the chanting into a conscious breathing practice.

To practice this way, simply watch the inhale and the exhale as you chant. As you focus on your breath, you are creating healing mindfulness within. If you are new to mantras, perhaps try using one powerful statement that you truly believe in, such as "I am sacred," saying the "I am" on the inhale and "sacred" on the exhale.

Try this: Inhale and silently say to yourself, "Open and expand." Then exhale and silently say to yourself, "Relax and let go." Do this as many times as you need to. By releasing positive, healing words into the universe, you are creating a positive, healing energy field around you.

Try sprinkling simple mantra breaths into your day as often as you can.

Singing

Why do so many women love singing Aretha Franklin's "Respect" at the top of their lungs after a breakup with someone they feel undervalued by? Because it's a cathartic form of altered breathing therapy. The songs you sing typically resonate with you, and by breathing out the song, you are also breathing out the emotions the song invokes.

Singing is a means of creating space and of letting go. And by listening to particular types of music, we can create a mood for ourselves. For example, when I listen to classical or instrumental music, I feel studious and creative. Inhaling this type of music sends a wave of sophistication and intellect through me. Whether you are singing to release emotions or listening to songs to create a feeling, do it mindfully, and you will feel the effects amplify.

Laughing

When you can't get the ketchup out of the bottle, what do you do? You shake it until it comes out. Laughter does the same for us: it shakes whatever feels immovable and loosens it. When we laugh from the belly, we release tension from the body.

The Dalai Lama refers to himself as "a professional laugher." Laughing can be a breathing meditation, albeit a nontraditional one. It is one of the greatest ways to release stuck emotions and resistances. Just try making yourself laugh for one minute, and then stop and mindfully observe the sensations you feel within the body afterward.

Exercising

When you exercise, you breathe harder and faster than normal. You heat your body, and the stuck or tense parts of you are able to move and shift. To make any form of exercise into a mindful alternative breathing practice, try to keep your conscious awareness on the breath throughout.

The Mindful Rituals

On average, you probably spend twenty minutes a day washing the dirt off your skin whenever you shower or take a bath. But how many minutes do you spend clearing the clutter from your mind?

The hardest part of a mindfulness practice is doing it consistently, as often as you possibly can. If your practice lacks consistency, the results will be hard to notice, and you will feel discouraged and practice less, not more. That's why a strict meditation retreat, like the one I attended in India, is a good place to start to practice: through this kind of experience you will immediately see the results.

But running off to a retreat isn't always possible for us, and it most certainly isn't necessary. In fact, when you start doing your meditation practice in your everyday life in your own home, you have the great advantage of integrating that skill into your daily routine right away.

I know how hard it is to dedicate time to just breathing and nothing else — trust me. I am not a monk; I have the same struggles and never-ending to-do lists that everyone else does. In many ways, creating spaciousness is the first thing you must do. If your excuse for not meditating is that you don't have the time, return back to your creating space rituals to see how you can create the time needed.

For years I gave myself strict rules for what style of meditation I should practice and for how long. I believed that meditation consisted of sitting for at least thirty minutes every day, cross-legged, while watching the natural breath. I felt guilty and gave myself a hard time when I didn't practice in this way. And I often didn't. This led me to more self-bullying... and less mindfulness.

When I switched to meditating for ten minutes three times a day, I found that I made it happen more frequently. Practicing in this way allowed me to sprinkle mindfulness throughout my day. I let my meditation practice become more fluid: I'd take ten minutes to focus on the breath while bathing, grab five minutes while waiting for a doctor's appointment, and take a few conscious breaths here and there while cooking. Suddenly, I felt more mindful on a regular basis, because I was creating more mindful moments each and every day.

After my son was born, I stopped sitting cross-legged altogether. My breathing practices started to happen when I was breastfeeding and putting him to sleep, usually while lying down. In fact, I believe that Kona, my son, is the greatest breath work teacher of my life, because he is the one who taught me to be less critical and strict about how I was practicing and to focus more on simply making it happen.

Now, most of the conscious breaths I take are integrated into my daily life as little sparkles of breathing awareness. While standing in line at the grocery store, cleaning the house, even working at my computer, I stop and consciously breathe to the count of ten. (I even stopped halfway through writing that sentence to sprinkle a little more presence into this moment!) Try it, right now, before you begin the next paragraph.

Discipline is training oneself to do something in a controlled and habitual way. Meditation is a discipline for changing the habitual patterns of your mind. What we are doing here is not striving to change or desperately trying to become something different, but simply learning skills and integrating them into our lives through disciplined practice.

On some days you will find it harder than others to come to your practice. I have discovered that these are the opportunistic moments to make the great breakthrough leaps in your mindfulness skills. Resolve to give these difficult days the most importance of all.

Remember that when you are meditating and the mind constantly wanders, as is its tendency, you are still developing mindfulness during your session. Try not to get discouraged. When you are counting your breaths and you lose count, you are still generating mindful concentration within your mind. If during your meditation your thoughts constantly flicker from your grocery list to your workweek ahead, you are still meditating and cultivating mindful awareness.

By returning to your breath with conscious awareness as often as you can, you are creating a habitual, disciplined pattern of presence in your life.

Create Your Mindfulness Rituals: Vinyasa Krama

Keep a few primary considerations in mind when creating your mindfulness rituals:

Time. How much time can you commit (without undue struggling) to your rituals? Remember, these are the steps for manifesting your dreams; they are important, but you also need to be realistic about what you are actually going to be able to do. Once you know exactly how much time you can dedicate to your mindfulness rituals, then it is time to curate them.

Practices. Think about which practices you'd like to include from each of the following categories.

- **Traditional meditation practices.** What breathing practices resonate with you the most? Are there one, two, or three particular practices that you feel drawn to? List a few breath work / meditation practices that you would like to start working with. Personally, I like to dedicate the first ten minutes or so of my mindfulness rituals to practicing natural breathing meditation, because it helps me ground into the present moment. Then I dedicate the next twenty minutes to scanning and mindfully breathing into all of the individual parts of my body. If I feel stressed or notice tension along the way, I give a little extra intentional conscious breath to those more stressed areas. If I notice I am feeling a certain way, I may integrate an altered breathing practicing into my daily yoga session.

  If you are not sure which traditional meditation practices to begin with, start with the first two breathing practices in this chapter, mindfulness of breathing and Zen breath counting, and then add ten rounds of bumblebee (brahmari) calming breaths at the end.

- **Unorthodox breathing practices.** Making the time to do more of what you love is the key to a happier life, but you can also do something that you find fun and that simultaneously develops your mindfulness, such as laughing, chanting, singing, or exercising. I end most meditations with some mantra breathing, taking a few rounds of breath to move a phrase within and outside of me.

  Now, list a few unorthodox ways you can integrate more conscious breaths into your life.

- **Additional practices.** Make note of any additional rituals you feel will benefit your mission to create more mindfulness in your life.

5

Developing Awareness

*Man's concept of his world built on the experience of the five senses
is no longer adequate and in many cases no longer valid.*

— SHAFICA KARAGULLA

D id you know that if you are quiet enough, you can actually hear your heart beating? And you can feel the waves
of blood ebbing and flowing through your fingers, even to the
point that you can take your own pulse from within, simply by
feeling for it.

In this chapter, you will learn how the yogis taught us to
feel the depths of ourselves, the parts of us we can't actually see.
In this stage, which the yogis call *pratyahara*, or "sense with-
drawal," we are learning (metaphorically) how to put our head
beneath the surface of our skin, the way we would use a pair
of swimmer's goggles to see beneath the surface of the ocean.
The tools the yogis offer us in this fifth step are the goggles to
see within ourselves.

I find the ocean to be one of the greatest metaphors for our

99

human body: its sensations, its waves and energies, its depths, the uncertainty of what lives within. What lies in the deepest parts of the oceans, no one knows. Similarly, most of us move through life feeling disconnected from the deepest parts of ourselves.

I have always been an avid ocean lover, swimming, sailing, and surfing in her mysteries every chance I get. I started dabbling in the ocean's soulful teachings at the age of twenty-five, when I first sailed. One day, while I was sitting in a riverside café in Río Dulce, Guatemala, I met a sailor looking for crew to help him sail his rather dilapidated boat to the Bay Islands of Honduras.

An hour later, we pulled the anchor and headed out to sea. This was the beginning of teachings with what is in my opinion Earth's greatest guru, the ocean. I was hooked; from then on, I had to be on the ocean.

For the next five years, in Alaska, I worked and lived on the ocean for months at a time. I spent three summer seasons as a wilderness guide from the bow of a sixty-foot steel fishing boat turned intimate liveaboard ship. I would guide tourists to see one of the most incredible places on Earth, Prince William Sound. From the boat, we would kayak, watch glaciers calve, admire breeching orcas, and explore uninhabited islands on a daily basis.

Traveling by ocean allows you to see things from an entirely different perspective. My time aboard boats taught me you can never take your eyes off of the ocean, or a surprise will come and throw everything into a reckless state of havoc. The ocean demands a sailor's undivided attention — constant mindful awareness.

The more time a sailor spends observing the ocean, the

more clarity and understanding she or he gains about how it works. Eventually, the sailor learns how to navigate storms and find safety in protective coves. The most experienced sailors in the world actually use windstorms and strong currents to their advantage, to sail further and faster, but they must spend time getting to know the ocean first, and then they understand how to use her energy for power.

My last day of work on the MV *Discovery* in Alaska was the same day I moved into my friend's yurt in the mountains. There I started dreaming of being near the ocean again, but this time to surf.

In the beginning surfing felt impossible. I was scared to go out into the wild waves and often left the water feeling rather defeated and looking like a drowned cat. Yet I always felt my time soaking in the ocean was sacred; something profound was happening when I was around her, and she continued to lure me back in different ways time and time again.

Each time I paddled out, I was learning a little more of how the ocean works. A storm far out at sea would send energy waves through her waters to me, somewhere on shore. And if I timed it just right, I was able to ride one of those little waves.

I may never truly know or see what lives in the deepest chasms of the ocean, but I do feel that I am connected with her the more I dive into the sea or float on her surface — as I experience how she functions and I play with her energy.

To see into the depths of ourselves, we must leave the safety of the shoreline and look within. It might be difficult or scary initially, but the first time you use your mindfulness to go within the skin of your body and simply feel, you start to understand not only the parts of the physical anatomy that you have never seen, like your kidneys and heart, but your energetic and conscious anatomy as well.

Feel Deeply

Feelings are not science based; they are phenomena happening within your body. Feelings are like rainbows: you might not be able to touch them, and they change as you move and grow, but they most certainly exist.

It took me nearly ten years to truly understand this fifth stage of yoga. Most of my yoga life, I was dedicated to a strict daily Mysore-style Ashtanga yoga practice — you know, the kind where you put your leg behind your head, contortionist style?

On most days, I did the same exact movement routine. I would also spend a little time meditating; I believed that if I did these two things enough, I would find the contentment, peace, and happiness I so desperately yearned for. Ironically, I was so inflexible with my daily yoga routine that I was actually building tension and resistance within my body rather than eliminating them. Clearly, this was not my path to contentment, even though my mind constantly told me it was.

Most of those years, I rarely stopped to listen for how I felt. Looking back on it, I see that so many clear intuitive messages were coming through, but I mostly ignored them. I had a plan, or so I thought. I kept all of those gut instincts and heartfelt dreams hidden away under my thick blanket of routine and predictability in order to stay comfortable and secure in what I knew.

I never saw the big picture of yoga. I didn't really understand how yoga worked as a comprehensive system. I studied with a lot of teachers, did countless trainings and courses, and read plenty of books, but I never clearly recognized yoga as a strategy — a system, if you will.

Now, I see it that way. And I realize that this step of the yoga process is the bridge, guiding us from the more outward aspects of yoga — the physical body and the mind —into our spiritual center, our inner world, our soul. We accomplish this by feeling.

The ancient yogis offered us pratyahara for learning to feel. This deep, meditative examination of one's inner self is exactly how the earliest sailors, astrologists, cosmologists, physicians, psychologists, and spiritual healers gained their knowledge. Much like our modern X-ray machines, pratyahara practices are techniques for seeing into the body in order to understand it.

This is how the first Portuguese explorers set sail for what was to them a new world despite being told the Earth was flat. This is how the yogis themselves came up with the system I am sharing with you here today. It is also how I came to write the book you are reading.

Our human bodies are dynamic and intricate. There is a depth to us that can be difficult to connect to without a conscious intention to do so. In the same way most choose to stay on the shorelines of the oceans, many people choose to stay on the surface of themselves, never taking the time to look deeply within and quite possibly never in their entire lives connecting with the meaning of life.

As Carl Jung explained, "I have found from experience that the basic psychological functions ... prove to be thinking, feeling, sensations, and intuition." There are differences among these layers of psychological functioning. Now you know how to identify all of these within yourself. Only by familiarizing yourself well with each of them, slowly over time, will you gain the keen awareness to notice just how different these styles of inner communication are and where they are stemming from. This is important, because when it comes to living a life of soulful purpose, you want to be sure you're making decisions and choices, not from thoughts, feelings, or sensations, but from your intuition.

Connecting with Your Superpowers

Essentially, the yogis teach us to become experts at ourselves. They want us to see ourselves for what we are. They begin with the obvious, the physical body and the breath, and then dive into the less visible and more felt mechanisms of our inner self. Once we begin to feel within, we discover layers of our existence still to be unpacked. You may feel emotional waves, body sensations, or energetic thicknesses in certain areas, as well as a felt sense of direction or clarity that lacks reasoning or logic.

In Alaska, I have a friend who lost his eyesight in an unfortunate run-in with a protective mama bear a few years back. Although he can no longer see, his other senses have become more powerful and acute since that day. Specifically, he has become an incredible listener. He can recognize my voice in a crowded room even if we haven't been together for years. It's absolutely mind-boggling. He has also become a remarkable musician in the time since he lost his eyesight.

As his example shows, by disconnecting from certain senses, your others become stronger. Furthermore, by closing yourself off to your physical senses — sight, smell, taste, hearing, and touch — your sixth sense, inner feeling, naturally grows stronger. The technique the yogis gave us for doing this is *pratyahara*, which literally means "gaining mastery over *ahara*, or external influences." This is precisely what we are working on here.

Pratyahara is a tool for connecting you to the intuitive parts of yourself so that you can know what they are communicating to you. Essentially, the more you learn to withdraw your mindfulness from the senses on the surface and allow your concentrated gaze to move within, the more you advance your skills of feeling into your inner self.

Albert Einstein claimed that most of his craziest ideas came to him intuitively, specifically when playing his beloved violin. In a letter to the great pioneer of musical education Shinichi Suzuki, Einstein shared with him that "the theory of relativity occurred to me by intuition." It was only after his intuition suggested something inside him that he would tirelessly work to prove these subconscious hunches to the scientific community in thoughts, logic, and words. In addition to realizing the groundbreaking theory of relativity, Einstein also introduced a new way to look at science when he said, "All great achievements of science must start from intuitive knowledge."

In my opinion, it is through this stage of moving within that yogis learn to perform miracles using their supernatural powers, which are called *siddhis*. Perhaps we could even say Einstein himself became so intuitive he created his own scholarly style of siddhi power.

Siddhi is a Sanskrit noun that can be translated as "perfection," "accomplishment," "attainment," "success," or "power." Siddhis arise when you are so aware and focused on what is happening within you, especially your intuition, that you gain incredible abilities and strength. This ability to focus intensely within is exactly how people like Wim Hof, "the Iceman," continue to break world records, over and over. They too have developed their own siddhi superpowers. Still to this day the highest ordained Tibetan monks use pratyahara and their own siddhis to find and appoint the next Dalai Lamas.

Another example of a dedicated pratyahara practitioner is the Vietnamese monk Thich Quang Duc. On June 11, 1963, as a form of political protest, Thich sat peacefully in Lotus Pose on a street corner in Saigon, Vietnam, as his entire body was engulfed in flames. Thich was completely in control of his mind. As his body burned to ashes, he sat there unmoving, never once opening his eyes, flinching in pain, or making a sound.

Siddhis do not appear in everyone. In fact, the yogis warned that these superpowers can actually be a distraction along one's spiritual path. I hope you don't see gaining siddhi superpowers as your goal but as an inspiration. When you fully familiarize yourself with your inner anatomy to the point of being intuitive, you will see that you already embody this sort of limitlessness — that you can do what once seemed impossible to your thinking mind. You start to understand the answer to the question "Who am I?"

Depths of Yourself Meditation

Take a moment now and slowly read through the imaginative meditation that follows. You can also record it and play it back to yourself.

Imagine yourself as a vast, open ocean. Imagine the depth

of your soul, like the deepest trenches of the ocean, completely unknown and unfathomable to the thinking mind. Now slowly float your way to the surface, feeling your skin. Feel the tingling sensations of your fingertips and the ends of your toes, like the waves we see lapping along the ocean's shoreline.

Put the book down for a moment and let the breath guide you between the shadowy, unknown waters at the depth of your core and the shoreline of your skin. Most of the turbulence of the ocean lives on its surface; the same is true of most of the turbulence within you. The deeper you go, the clearer and calmer everything becomes.

Let your mindful concentration move through the spaciousness within you and allow yourself to feel into this depth a little more profoundly with each breath. While it is easy to walk along the shoreline for one's entire life, it takes courage to dive headfirst into the depths of the sea and to feel around for what lives there. Similarly, it takes courage to dive into the hidden depths of yourself, because you will find things that might make you want to turn away. Even though humans have now been to the moon, we have yet to go to the bottoms of our oceans.

Simply sit here and be with this depth. Feel into it. Observe. Just be with whatever arises within. Be quiet and still, continuously observing without judgment, listening intently. From this place, when an intuitive ping comes alive within you, you will feel it.

Stay here as long as you would like. Being in this space and simply observing what is happening within is the entire purpose of our feeling practices. From this place, you will feel your intuition bubbling to the surface.

The Feeling Practices

How do you teach someone to feel? How do you explain to someone the way to move into their depth, the subconscious parts of themself?

The sixteenth-century Hindu mystic poet Mirabai was perhaps the most renowned woman poet saint of India. Mirabai wrote, "In my travels I spent time with a great yogi. / Once he said to me, / Become so still you hear the blood flowing / through your veins. One night as I sat in quiet, / I seemed on the verge of entering a world inside so vast / I know it is the source of / all of / us." This is how we will learn to feel, by quietly observing our innate self, full of subtle feelings.

The feeling practices are yogic techniques to help you feel more deeply and see into who you truly are, deep down in your soul. The awakened yogis of the past gave us practices of relaxation, mindful awareness, and analytical meditation to help us see what lies beneath the body's skin layer. These practices will guide you to see all the things — organs, blood, energy, meridian lines, chakras, and conscious layers — that make up your humanness. They guide you into the powerful inner architecture of the self, leading you to none other than your soul's core.

You will learn to feel yourself through different lenses: emotionally, energetically, and consciously. The feeling practices are explorations into the unknown, so go into them with a beginner's mind.

For many years, two of the feeling practices, chakra-balancing meditations and aura-layer visualizations, felt exotic and far-fetched to me. Perhaps I wasn't quite ready for them yet. Years later, when I came back to these same practices with greater mindful sensitivity, I started to sense my anatomical body as something other than mere tissues and organs — as something vast, unscientific, and utterly mystical.

Feeling practices should begin with a mindfulness practice, because this relaxes the body and a relaxed body is imperative if you want to move deep within. We don't jump right into a wild, raging ocean; we wait for the waters of the sea to calm, and then we go in.

A natural by-product of mindfulness is relaxation. Without even trying, the body and the mind relax as you become more mindful. Without first embodying the skill of mindfulness, it is impossible to truly embody the skill of feeling.

In just a few short minutes of practicing mindful meditation, your nervous system moves into a parasympathetic stress response, otherwise known as "rest and digest." Your heart rate slows down, your breathing rate slows, your thoughts slow, and the physical body naturally softens. In other words, walls are coming down around you. Once your body is completely soft and relaxed, it feels safe, even if a bit vulnerable. It can then open. When this happens, you are ripe for feeling into your own depths.

Some yogis have learned to relax so deeply that they cease to be conscious of their physical bodies at all, like the old Indian teacher at my first meditation retreat, who sat for hours on end without ever moving his legs from his meditation position. When you enter this deeper part of your consciousness, you enable yourself to dive into your juicy, soulful core, into the depths of yourself.

There are many ways to start exploring your inner world. I have simplified the expansive world of pratyahara practices down to three of my personal favorites: (1) yoga nidra; (2) energy meditations; and (3) nada yoga. I will also share some of my favorite unorthodox methods for moving within.

We will start our journey into the inner world by first meditating on the five layers of consciousness as explained in yogic texts. Through my practices of yoga nidra, I learned about the layers of our consciousness, called "sheaths." These resemble the layers of an onion, each one protecting the others beneath. I learned that by relaxing each of these layers in turn, I could sense all the way down to my subconscious roots, deeply releasing my entire body.

Next, we will explore the feelings of energies by familiarizing ourselves with the energy centers and lines that run through the body as explained in Taoism, Traditional Chinese Medicine, Tibetan Buddhism, and Ayurveda. When I started focusing my meditative observation on my energetic body, I began to understand that the fast and slow waves of energies I felt as sensations were a side effect of the deeper energies moving through me.

Finally, we will talk about nada yoga, the yoga of sound. I found that meditating with musical instruments, sound baths, chanting, prayer, and mantras enabled me to feel the slightest sound waves vibrating deep inside me. This resonated strongly with me, and I found myself leaning toward nada yoga for my feeling practices turned rituals, because listening to music has always been deeply enjoyable to me and now I was using it to heal.

In the same way that in previous chapters we retrained the mind to become more focused by creating our spaciousness and mindfulness rituals, now we learn to take that focus and start to turn it within. The yogis called this process *svadhyaya,* meaning "self-inquiry." It is one of the five values — (the niyamas we discussed in chapter 1) — that they suggested we diligently direct ourselves toward.

These suggested practices for feeling are helpful to get you started, but know that the feeling practices are limitless.

Sitting with strong emotions, such as grief and heartbreak, also teaches us to feel. Perhaps strong life emotions exist simply so that we can connect with our soul.

Yoga Nidra and the Conscious Layers

The yogis teach us that there are layers of consciousness, like an onion, wrapped around you. As you familiarize yourself with these, you learn to relax them so you can continue moving deeper into the soulful layers beneath.

When I was three months pregnant, I signed up for an iRest yoga nidra training taught by psychologist Richard Miller. I spent a week on the Gold Coast of Australia with a group of psychologists — and a few social workers and yoga teachers mixed in — learning how to systematically relax my body, part by part, in order to feel what lay beneath the surface.

In many ways, yoga nidra is similar to hypnosis; they both guide you to relax everything on the surface, so you can feel the strong impulses bubbling up through each of the layers into your conscious awareness. Another beautiful aspect of the yoga nidra process is that you can actually send messages right into the subconscious self. Through yoga nidra, you learn to let go and to create in the same breath, without even trying — it just happens.

Through this intensive study into myself while I was, shall I say, heavily spacious in my belly, I heard loud and clear messages. First I felt a strong ping to write a book. I didn't take the message completely seriously, but with each additional session, the message continued and grew clearer: I was to write a book about intuition, manifestation, and the process of yoga.

Suddenly, just like Dorothy in *The Wizard of Oz*, I saw my

own unique yellow brick road opening before me, taking me to where I wanted to go and toward who I wanted to become. With each step I took forward, the road became more defined. For the first time in my life, I felt I was making decisions from my internal sixth sense rather than from the logistical ideal-isms of my logical mind. It felt like I was gaining momentum in life simply by floating, not driving. Some might call what I experienced an epiphany.

I didn't force myself to write when anxious, because that would have been taking action from my logical mind telling me, "You have a deadline, so keep working until it is done." Instead, a burst of inspiring ideas and examples would come to me when I rested, while doing my yoga nidra meditations, so I started writing from that space. I felt that I was channeling something, much in the way Einstein described.

Suddenly nothing felt forced; writing and explaining came with a natural ease, an alignment and a flow. At first, this flow applied only to my writing. In time, however, I further developed this approach toward how I live — in each moment, led by the way I feel, forcing nothing. Yoga nidra meditations have shown me how to do all of these things.

The five layers of your consciousness in traditional yogic texts are (in order):

1. *Annamaya kosha:* physical body sensations
2. *Pranayama kosha:* breath and energy
3. *Manomaya kosha:* emotions
4. *Vijnanamaya kosha:* intellect, thoughts, and beliefs
5. *Anandamaya kosha:* joy and love

A guided yoga nidra practice almost always begins with the intention to relax the body, starting with the outermost physical layer, *annamaya kosha*. This is the material layer made up of our physical sensations, such as pain, tickling, warmth, sweating, and coolness on the skin and in the muscles. You activate this layer of consciousness when practicing asana or when you feel pain within the body.

Once the physical outer body is calm and relaxed, you will start to feel into the layer beneath it. As you watch the sensations of the chest rising and falling while you breathe, you may awaken to the softer, subtler layer just below, the breath and energy layer, *pranayama kosha*. When we rest and relax the mind on the breath, it doesn't take long for emotions and memories to bubble up. This happens because you are starting to sense your feelings layer, *manomaya kosha*. With practice, you will learn to soften and relax and stay equanimous to the comings and goings in this feelings layer. Then you can move into the layer of your intellectual wisdom, *vijnanamaya kosha*.

All these layers cover the most subconscious layer of all: our soulful center. This is where our soul's purpose and guidance speak to us from. This is where the whispers you feel in the other layers of your consciousness come from. This is why your wisdom and emotions, breath and outer sensations can be activated from the intuition — because it lives beneath them all.

As you learn to feel and hear your intuition, you open your awareness to the peaceful, joyful, loving home base of you, *anandamaya kosha*, where the soul lives within you. This is the final layer. The Tibetan Buddhists often refer to this realm as emptiness, because it is vast and infinite in possibilities.

You will know when you have touched into this core layer because it gives off an amazing calm, settled, and relaxed feeling. When we are in touch with this deepest layer of ourselves, our soul layer, we can spread its illumination into all the other layers of our consciousness, thus becoming more soulful.

This is why many spiritual teachers tell us our true nature is calm and at peace — because it is. The core of you is loving, generous, warm, and joyful. Connecting with this layer offers us incredible self-worth and confidence, because we see for ourselves that we are a soul living in a human body, and seeing that with your own mind helps you realize just how magical you are.

While in some ways the five layers are distinct, they are also clearly interconnected. For example, when your thoughts are of a loved one who has passed away and the emotion of grief fills your mind, you will feel this as heaviness in the lungs and possibly experience difficulty breathing. Or perhaps if you remember the first time you fell in love you may feel butterflies in your belly.

I love yoga nidra because it gets you right into the good stuff, your true nature. This meditation technique is powerful for helping you find your answers to questions such as "Who am I?," "Why am I?," "What is the purpose of this life?," and "What is enlightenment?" You are able to hear your dreams, and if you relax even more, you learn how your soul is guiding you to create those dreams. It's all there, just waiting to be explored.

During a yoga nidra meditation, as the entire body relaxes and moves into a slightly hypnotic state, you guide your awareness closer to the soulful golden nectar that lies beneath each of the layers. When it comes to intuition, I believe yoga nidra is one of the most beneficial practices of all. By combining intentionality, mindful meditation, deep relaxation, and in-depth awareness, you gain direct access to your soul.

In fact, there are stories from people who have had comas

and near-death experiences, unconsciously released all tension and resistance within the body, and returned to life with an understanding of this deep, subconscious state of soulfulness.

One of my favorite examples is in the writings of Eben Alexander, a contemporary neuroscientist who was in a coma for a week and was clinically determined to be brain-dead. Alexander came out of his coma with an entire book of explanations and realizations about consciousness, *Proof of Heaven*, which became a bestseller. "During my seven days of coma, I not only remained fully conscious but journeyed to a stunning world of beauty and peace and unconditional love," he wrote. "I underwent the most staggering experience of my life, my consciousness traveling to another level."

Feeling your soul with your human body is one of the most mind-opening moments for any spiritual seeker. Now that you understand the layers of your consciousness, it's time to lie back and simply focus your concentrated awareness within in order to start to live these concepts inside yourself, as firsthand experience.

Yoga Nidra Script: A Journey through the Five Koshas

You can read this meditation here or record it on your phone to listen to later.

Take the posture of Shavasana, lying down on your back with your arms resting to the sides of your body, palms facing upward. Relax your legs and hips and allow the feet to fall out to the sides. You can place a pillow beneath your head and/or a bolster under your knees to take pressure off your lower back. Make yourself as comfortable as you possibly can. Then ask yourself how you can become 10 percent more comfortable, and move into that.

Gently close your eyes and settle your mind on the breath. During the practice of yoga nidra, it is important to remain still for the duration in order for your awareness to turn fully inward. If you feel discomfort arising, let it be part of the experience, observing it and noticing how it functions within the body. Change your position only when absolutely necessary. Otherwise, simply observe without judgment but with pure awareness.

If at any time during this practice you are overwhelmed with emotions or past traumas, you can bring your mind to a place or person who gives you a feeling of peace and calm. Take a moment now to make a mental note of an inner resource you can call up whenever you need to calm yourself down.

Now, let the practice of yoga nidra begin. Let my words become your own and allow this journey to guide your awareness, illuminating the many different parts of yourself with mindful concentration.

Before we begin scanning through the body, let us create a soulful intention for this practice, called a *sankalpa*. A sankalpa is a heartfelt desire or wish. Always state your sankalpa as an "I am" statement, as fact in the present moment. If you want more happiness, your sankalpa would be "I am happy." If you want to feel calmer and more at peace, your sankalpa would be "I am calm and at peace." Take a moment now to create an "I am..." sankalpa in your practice.

State your personalized sankalpa statement now. You can repeat it a few times if you would like. As we relax throughout the meditation, this heartfelt intention will seep down into our relaxed subconscious body, like a seed being planted in fertile, aerated soil. Now we are ready to bring our conscious awareness to the physical layer of the body. Observe the sensations happening right now in your physical body. Bring your attention to rest lightly on the skin of your face. Allow your features and expressions to become neutral, soft, and tender. Feel the skin of your forehead and watch the tension naturally fall away as you breathe into this place. Let the space between the eyebrows expand from the center to the periphery, moving your attention along the eyebrows to your temples. Slowly draw a line from your temples to your ears. Observe the outer architecture of your ears and then follow the ear canals into the space between the inner ears, into the inner brain.

Observe the brain from the inside looking out; observe the inner walls of your skull. Now pull your concentration into your mouth. Feel the tongue, teeth, top jaw, and bottom jaw. Allow your lower jaw to hang loose at the hinge joint and observe the point where the jaws connect.

Move your attention down into your throat, through the neck, feeling the muscles running up and down the neck into the collarbone and shoulders. Let your awareness flow down the arms into the upper arms, elbows, lower arms, palms, and fingers. Return back up the arms and into your heart, in the center of your chest. Be here, in the heart, completely. Breathe into the heart, feeling the ribs moving with each inhale and exhale. Then slide your awareness down your spine, vertebrae by vertebrae. Bring your awareness into your belly, down into the pelvic girdle. Feel where the hips attach to the pelvis and then guide your awareness down your legs into your thighs, knees, shins, ankles, tops of the feet, soles of the feet, and each of your toes.

Now, in your own time, move back up through these body parts, using your mind as a flashlight, illuminating each part, but keeping your attention constantly moving. Be aware of all that is now present in your awareness. Experience yourself as the field of awareness in which everything is coming and going.

Become aware of the body breathing. Feel the flow of the breath as sensation in the nostrils. As you inhale, sense the abdomen gently rising as breath flows in. Exhale, feeling the breath flowing out. No need to change anything — just notice how the body breathes naturally and rhythmically. Inhale, abdomen rising. Exhale, abdomen releasing. Sense the body breathing itself; simply observe.

Now bring your attention to feelings that are present throughout the body, such as warmth or coolness. Do you observe any heaviness? Now look for the opposite of heaviness. Do you observe areas of lightness? Where can you feel comfort? Where is there discomfort? Allow whatever feelings are inside you to appear. If no feelings are present, as may happen, simply welcome whatever is present. Now, welcome both opposites of feeling into the body at the same time. Simply observe both simultaneously.

Now bring your attention to an emotion presently in your body or one that you are working with in your life. You can recall a memory that invites a particular emotion into your body, welcoming the emotion as sensation. Invite this emotion to unfold fully as a sensation in the body. If no emotion is present, be with that. Simply welcome whatever is present. Let your awareness move to where you feel this emotion within your body. Are there thoughts, images, or memories that arise along with this emotion? Take your time.

Then invite the opposite emotion to unfold within you. Feel it. Are there thoughts, images, or memories that arise with this emotion? And now invite both emotions to flow within you. Experience how you feel these emotions in the sensations of the body.

Now, bring your attention to a thought or belief presently in your body or one that you are working with in life. If a belief is present, where does it sit within you? Where do you feel it? What sensations does it come with? Notice any sensations, emotions, or thoughts that accompany it. And then invite an opposite thought or belief into yourself. Where does this belief sit? Where do you feel it? What sensations does it come with?

Notice any thoughts that may appear when you invite this belief to be observed. Feel space slightly outside your skin. Do you sense anything here? Do you notice the layer of your skin separating the inside of you from the outside?

Be in this field of awareness where everything is arising and passing away and ask yourself, *Is there a periphery to it? Is there a beginning or an end?* Simply observe. Welcome whatever emerges just as it is.

Now, imagine bliss. Immense inner bliss, like a smile radiating from deep within. Feel the warmth of love in your heart. Bring your awareness to the fact that everything is okay right here, right now. You are simply watching as thoughts, emotions, and sensations shift and reshape within you, constantly ebbing and flowing.

Feel life moving within you. Dissolve into this pure awareness, open and spacious, everything coming and going, and simply be with whatever is.

Surrender to being with everything just as it is. With yourself just as you are.

Now bring your awareness back to the breath, easy and rhythmic, and recall your sankalpa. Feel your sankalpa resonate through the sensations of the body, now alive in your consciousness. And experience your sankalpa as an accomplished fact. How does that feel?

Now, slowly start to emerge back into the world outside your personal awareness. Hear the sounds in the room. Open your eyes and look at what is outside you. Take this moment to feel yourself as this timeless, indestructible, open, and spacious body of awareness in which everything is constantly unfolding. And slowly, in your own time, come back to your open-eyed, alert sense of self.

Energy Meditations and the Energetic Body

When someone says, "I love your energy," what does that actually mean? I believe what most people are referring to when they use the word *energy* are the feeling-based phenomena emanating from within you.

Taoists see the universe as a great conduit of energy. Energy makes the planets spin. Energy makes your heart beat. Energy is the magical ingredient responsible for manifestation in all forms, yet many know little about it because of its intangible nature.

Energy is the vibratory nature of feeling-based phenomena. The Taoist word for energy is *qi*. *Qi* can be translated as "breath," "air," or "gas" and is the life force that animates all forms. Energy is how the material world moves. The Taoists call our energy centers *dan tians* and our energy channels, *meridians*.

In Hinduism, energy is called *shakti*. Hindus revere shakti as divine and believe it is what moves the entire universe and cosmos. Yogis believe that energy flows through the body via our *chakras*, or energy centers, and our *nadis*, or energy channels.

The chakra system is a way of simplifying a complex energetic body organization into a few main centers. Traditional writings mention 88,000 chakras. When narrowed down to the 40 main chakra centers, these are referred to as *marma points* in Ayurveda and *acupoints* in Traditional Chinese Medicine.

Energy is what creates life and sustains it. When all energy leaves the body, the heart stops beating, and the breath stops flowing; the body dies. The basis of all medicine in most of Asia is energy and how it moves.

In the same way that clogged arteries can cause heart attacks and strokes, energy in the body can become stagnant and blocked, causing disease and disturbances to your health and happiness. In Ayurveda, the yogic science of health, as well as in Traditional Chinese Medicine, energy is often described as being thick and grounded, fast and airy, or hot and fiery. By understanding the energy within a person, the health practitioners are able to help balance and heal it.

Taoist philosophy explains that people can move qi in the body by using the power of the concentrated mind. We are not necessarily forcing energy to move, but simply opening the mind enough for the energy to flow with more ease. In this way, energy meditations are similar to yoga nidra: the intention is to relax through mindfulness.

By taking the time each day to focus on your energetic body, you start to feel energies moving within you. For now, let's begin these practices by simply awakening our consciousness to the feelings of the energies in your body, not necessarily doing anything with them, but just becoming aware of them.

I have found that anxiety has a certain busy energy feeling to it that I can experience as thick and fast in the chest. I often feel sadness as a heavy and lethargic weight in the area around my heart. And bliss feels like open expansion and lightness all over the body.

This is why energy meditations are a great option for learning to feel. The yogis believed that we can only feel shakti, our energies, when we are awakened to it. They believe that only when we start to understand energy can we start to understand spirituality.

The ultimate intention of an energy practice is to feel what is happening within you below the surface. At first you may choose just to learn the energetic anatomy by practicing chakra, meridian, or dan tian meditations. As you become familiar with your energetic body, you can then intuitively focus your mindful awareness into particular parts of the body or specific energetic centers, which as you know by now will relax them.

With practice, you will start to see that these are the same energies that animate the world and cosmos around you. This is precisely what astrologists do. After thousands of years of energy observation and research, they have found that certain energies have a tendency to arise when the sun, moon, stars, and planets are situated in a particular way. For example, energy sensitivity is often amplified when the moon is full. A strong Libra moon will amplify a sense of balance in your emotional body, because the sign of Libra tends to bring balancing energies and the moon tends to affect our emotional body. Likewise, a Virgo moon can make us feel busier and detail oriented, the qualities of the Virgo sign.

There are endless avenues of energy that you can explore within yourself. Thousands of books, meditations, and practices exist for connecting you with your energetic body. Hindus believe that all you have to do is awaken your shakti, and everything else will start to unfold on its own.

Whether you are well practiced at feeling into your energetic body or a beginner, we practice in the same way. We simply create space by moving into a meditation and observe what is there.

A Chakra Meditation

Chakra is an ancient Sanskrit word that translates to "wheel." Our life force, or *prana*, that moves inside the body is connected to seven energy centers. They begin at the base of the spine and extend to the top of the head. When the chakras are unbalanced or closed tight, we might have health difficulties. So we will begin by moving through each chakra, bringing our energy and awareness to each of these places in turn before moving on to the next.

By bringing our energy to each chakra, we allow it to open, balance, and heal. Let us begin by coming to a comfortable meditation position. Take a few moments to sit quietly and calm the mind by following the breath in and out. Inhaling, lift the spine, letting the oxygen flow through the spinal cord. Exhale and let any tension or tightness flow out of the body.

As you inhale, imagine a channel running from the crown of your head to the tip of your tailbone. Breathe and continue moving your awareness up and down this channel. Inhale, create space, and exhale, observing whatever arises in your awareness.

Continue breathing in and out naturally. Then bring your awareness to the very base of the spine near your tailbone. This is your first or root chakra, called *muladhara*. Imagine a bright red light here just above the anus and the perineum. The root chakra is believed to be where we connect to our human experience. When we feel we need more — love, money, and/or productivity — to survive, we have an overactive root chakra, which can cause anxiety and jitteriness. Allow this red light to shine through the root chakra, balancing it. You may say, "I am safe" or "I am grounded" here. Allow the survival instinct that flows from this energy center to relax.

Now let the red light at the base of your spine travel to just below your belly button and transform into an orange color. *Svadhisthana*, the sacral chakra, is the energy center that is home to your creative life force. It is this chakra that helps us enjoy our life here on Earth, taking pleasure in such things as sex, good food, and creative activities. When our second chakra is out of balance, we find ourselves craving things that aren't good for us, which can lead to addictions and obesity. Imagine the orange light penetrating this area of the body and harmonizing it. You may say, "I am creating my life" and "I am happy" here.

Let this orange light fade into a yellow light that begins at your belly button and extends up to your breastbone, where your ribs connect in your chest. This is the third chakra, the *manipura* or solar plexus chakra. This chakra is where your self-confidence, identity, and personal power live. Our solar plexus is the seat of our intuition; our inner voice speaks to us through our gut. When your solar plexus is out of balance, you may feel like you don't belong or don't have a purpose, you may lack confidence, or you may be angry. Allow that yellow light to shine through this region, lighting up your entire third chakra. You may say, "I am living my purpose" or "I am guided by my intuition" here.

From the solar plexus, move up to the area of the heart as the yellow transforms into a radiant green. This is the fourth chakra, the *anahata* or heart chakra. The chakra is located right over your heart and radiates down to your breastbone and up to your throat. The anahata chakra is where your love, compassion, and kindness are empowered. This can be love for yourself as well as love for others. Imagine the bright green light shining on every cell of your heart, and say, "I am love," "I love others," "I am loving-kindness," or "I am a compassionate being." As you inhale, allow your heart and chest to open more, spreading the green light deeper into that space. As you exhale, allow that love and compassion to move down through the other three chakras below.

Now inhale and allow the green light to turn into a blue light as it moves into your throat, a blue light shining between your collarbones and up to the center of your brow, between your eyes. This is the fifth chakra, the throat chakra, called *vishuddha*. Here in this energetic center, you are given a voice to speak your truth. This chakra works closely with your heart chakra and stems from the feelings of love, worth, and confidence you have in yourself. Vishuddha powers your ability to speak your truth, proud and unafraid. When this chakra is in balance, you speak in a way that enlightens and inspires those around you. You may choose to say here, "I speak my truth" and "I have a beautiful message to share."

Allow the blue color in your throat to move up to your third eye, where a bright indigo light shines. The third eye is located between your eyebrows and radiates down to your mouth and up to the top of your head. This is your *ajna* chakra, your sixth chakra, which opens your mind to information that comes from beyond the material world and the five senses. It is here that we may sense extrasensory perception, intuition, or psychic energy. A few inches inside the brain from this point lives your pineal gland, which takes in light. It is responsible for helping you feel awake in the day and sleepy at night. The pineal gland gives your brain more information than the five senses. The best thing you can do to harmonize this chakra is to devote quiet solitary time to meditation in order for it to relax and reset.

As you move the indigo light at your third eye up to the crown of your head, allow it to transform into a bright, white, shining light. This is your seventh chakra, the crown chakra, or *sahasrara*. The crown chakra center radiates from the top of your head down in between your eyes and extends infinitely upward and outward, connecting you to the energy of the rest of the universe. The only way to balance this chakra is to balance all the other six chakras. By meditating, connecting to your soul and spirit, and understanding the layers of your consciousness, you can balance your entire chakra body.

Now take a few moments to move these areas of the body and observe what you feel in each. Bring your awareness to what you are feeling in each area and be with it. When you feel ready, in your own time, return to your eyes-open, alert state of consciousness.

Nada Yoga and Vibrational Feeling

When you practice sound healing, you are feeling the vibrations and resonances of sound inside the body. *Nada* translates to "vibrations," and when you are doing nada yoga, you are using these vibrations to feel within yourself. Prayer, mantra singing and chanting, and musical instrument meditations are some types of sound healing practices.

Hindus, Muslims, Catholics, and Buddhists all chant mantras often. The Christian New Testament claims that "in the beginning there was the Word." Hinduism states that the universe began with one cosmic vibrational sound, "om," which created all matter and life as we know it. Sound is yet another form of energy, and we can use it to help us connect with the energy within ourselves.

Once, I took a road trip through Tibet, and my driver literally chanted the entire time for ten days. Tibetan chants take on a low, guttural tone that moves through the body as vibration. By the end of that journey, I felt a spacious freedom despite the fact that I had just spent ten days in a car. I believe those Tibetan chants vibrated the energy within me, healing me, even though I had no idea how at the time.

Unorthodox Methods for Feeling

In modern-day society, it is a common life tactic for people to stay busy so they can avoid processing hard emotions, as it can be incredibly painful to face them. Processing moments in life involves feeling what is there and finding an acceptance of it. This is why grief, heartbreak, and sadness are often our greatest spiritual learning experiences: because they force us to do the work of feeling what we might otherwise avoid.

In 2020, when the world shut down because of the Covid-19 pandemic, many of us for the first time found ourselves unable to travel or even to work. I am sure many people would agree that this year was very much centered around learning to sit and be with ourselves without our everyday distractions — as hard as it might have been at times and as much as we wanted to escape it, as we always have in the past.

If you can learn to simply be with the feelings currently within you, resting in them to the point of acceptance, you will discover an immense opportunity for spiritual growth. In the same way our mindfulness practices teach us that our thoughts come and go, we can start to observe that our feelings are always coming and going as well. And we can become skilled at not reacting to them.

Relaxing into and exploring yourself may involve seeing old wounds and pains that still live inside you, but if you can observe and learn to accept them, they too will pass. Moments of sadness and suffering fuel our personal growth. As we come to see life with a more truthful understanding, we change the way we live.

When we understand our true nature — which is exactly what these feeling practices are showing us — we start doing the things that make us happy and fulfilled on the inside and lessen our striving to become something we feel external pressure to be. Without even realizing it, we become more intuitive and soul driven.

It was the death of my college boyfriend that introduced me to grief. Before that moment I wanted to be a wartime journalist, because I felt that would be exciting and people would respect me. The minute grief took over, my focus shifted completely to the warlike feelings living within me. Suddenly, I understood how my inner pain and suffering were somehow connecting me to the spiritual. I learned to feel my way through the darkness, observing it and letting it pass through me. In the space that remained, I could hear my intuition more loudly than before.

When life feels difficult, feel into that — don't cringe from it or avoid it. This is your soul teaching you how to feel at the deepest of levels, the soul level. Life is meant to be felt, because feelings are what drive us toward truth.

Relax

I can't say it enough: the more you relax, the more you will feel without reacting to what arises. Anything that is intensely relaxing can help you feel more deeply: Reiki treatments, massages, floating in a pool, lying on a beach, walking, running. As you engage in any relaxation activity, simply observe the feelings moving through you without reacting to them. Ask yourself, *What relaxes me?*

A Candle Meditation

Once at an ashram in Lonavala, India, my ninety-year-old yoga teacher taught me a type of meditation using a candle as the object of my meditation practice. He told me, "This will help you connect to your intuition."

Yogis have used *trataka* meditation — single-pointed concentration on a candle flame — for centuries to tap into the subconscious. Fire has been a central element in most spiritual rituals and gatherings throughout history. Native Americans and tribal African peoples often ceremonially drum and dance around the fire (a form of nada yoga). Similarly, Catholics, Jews, and Buddhists light candles as part of their rituals.

Fire is a common symbol used for alchemy and transformation. Hindus believe that fire is the messenger between the human and the divine. Try this candle meditation and see if it resonates with you.

Light a candle, turn off the lights in the room, and sit a few feet away. Watch the flame moving, staying mindfully focused. Keep your eyes open, attempting not to blink, until tears develop. Then close your eyes and lie comfortably on the floor, safely away from the candle. Watch the flame imprint that stays in your mind for as long as you can.

Lie here as long as you like. You can repeat the process several times if you wish, making sure to take space between each round to feel for what comes up.

Journaling

Journaling has always been a way for me not only to express how I am feeling but to discover what my intuition is asking of me.

When you write by hand, your thoughts slow down; you simply cannot write as fast as you can think. When I journal, I fill the blank pages with musings on life, quotes, doodles, ideas, and whatever else I am moved to write down. Creative journaling is a way to see, in clear black and white, a manifestation of what you are feeling.

Your soulful dreams come only when they are felt intuitively, from within. Keep notes of the dreams that come up and notice if any repeat.

Once again, the practices for learning to feel are limitless. Make an intention to stop and feel more, and you are sure to reap the benefits.

The Feeling Rituals

You are always full of feelings. They are there inside of you every moment of every day. By creating a daily ritual for taking notice of what's going on inside, you create a habit of feeling.

My journey to becoming intuitive looked something like this: During the quiet space of meditative breathing or during a practice dedicated to feeling, I received epiphanies, hunches, pings, dreams. These ideas were so clear and powerful there was no confusing them with distracting thoughts, sensations, or emotions. My dreams became evident while I engaged in the feeling practices.

You cannot scientifically prove how much a mother loves a child, but we all know how much love she feels because we can sense it. As you study the architecture of the unseen parts of the body, you will better understand the ethereal elements within you and the mysterious ways these elements exist in the universe. In other words, the more you understand about the energy living within you, the more you understand the energy of the field surrounding you.

The greatest technique for becoming intuitive is to stop and feel. This is why creating and practicing your own feeling rituals is such an important process to commit to if you want to learn what your soul is asking of you. This will enable you to start to tap into your own unique superpowers and to make your dreams into your reality.

Create Your Feeling Rituals: Vinyasa Krama

Here are a few primary considerations to keep in mind when creating your feeling rituals.

Time. How much time can you commit (without struggling) to your feeling rituals? Remember, these rituals are the key steps for getting to know your dreams, but you also should be realistic about what you are actually going to commit to. Once you are sure about how much time you can dedicate to your feeling rituals, then it is time to curate them and create a sequence of this length to use every day.

Relaxation. It is easier to feel deeply when the physical body and the mind are relaxed. Always begin your feeling rituals with a relaxation practice. What is the most efficient practice that relaxes you? How do you unwind? List ways you can dedicate time to relaxing more each and every day. If you aren't sure where to start, begin with yoga nidra or progressive relaxation meditations every day for two weeks.

Feeling. Ask yourself this: What is the best way for you to really stop and look into how you are feeling? What feeling practices resonate with you the most? Are there one, two, or three particular practices that help you understand what you are feeling more clearly? A few ideas for your feeling rituals are daily meditation, a weekly yoga nidra, or ten minutes daily dedicated solely to stopping whatever you are doing and simply feeling.

Journaling. Journaling makes the mind spacious and focused for diving into your feelings. It doesn't necessarily need to be a part of your rituals, but in the beginning, it helps to include it because it will create a healthy habit of turning to your journal when expressing your feelings. You will be able to look back and see what was happening within by reviewing your mindful feeling-based writings.

Additional practices. Add any additional rituals you think will benefit your mission of feeling more deeply in your everyday life. If any extra techniques come to mind that support your ability to feel, incorporate them into your rituals.

6

The Intuition Rituals

Knowing how you actually want to feel is the most potent form
of clarity that you can have. Generating those feelings is the most
powerfully creative thing you can do in your life.

— Danielle LaPorte

In this chapter, I will guide you to create your own road map that will help you piece together all the little steps necessary to arrive at your big dream. These intuition rituals will help you see the larger picture. Until you are clear on what you passionately want and what your soul is asking from you, it will be impossible to feel you are living your purpose.

When I sat in the spaciousness of my friend's yurt deep in the mountains that cold Alaska winter, I had a resounding urge to surf. A few months later, while I was in Sri Lanka learning to surf, I had another urge to start teaching yoga. This whisper took me to Bali. In Bali, I met a man who soon became my husband and brought me my son, Kona.

Pregnant with Kona, I spent six months lying and listening

to yoga nidra relaxation practices. That was when I felt the strongest urge of all, to write this book. I didn't know what I would write about, and I certainly had never written a book before, but now I knew how to listen to my soul. All the guidance I needed was there inside me. I found that when I stuck to my spaciousness, mindfulness, and feeling rituals to stay connected to that inner voice, all the details of my life seemed to sort themselves out. The more I allowed my intuition to guide me, the more I felt I was surrendering to life rather than controlling it.

Your intuition is speaking to you all the time, but unless you have a consistent practice of mindfully feeling into the spaciousness, you will miss its messages altogether. If you can't feel for your intuition, you won't understand your purpose, and your life will feel it lacks meaning.

I urge you to practice these rituals with diligence. Your intuition rituals offer you an organized plan to find answers to what your soul is asking from you. Get clear on this before moving on.

Remember, not once in this book have I suggested that you sit and think about the question "What are my dreams?" Rather, I gave you three skills to develop in your life —spaciousness, mindfulness, and feeling awareness — and the practices to make them come alive within you. Without these three skills, you can search forever to no avail.

Your Intention Defines Your Path: Sadhana, Part I

The ancient yogis called one's daily yoga ritual *sadhana*. Sadhana is a discipline and dedicated practice in pursuit of a goal. Your daily sadhana practice is the series of action steps you create — the rituals — to help you grow in the exact ways you want and need to. In this book, I guide you to create two sadhana practices: your intuition rituals (in this chapter) and your manifestation rituals (in chapter 9). Your intuition rituals are how you will clarify your dreams, and your manifestation rituals are how you will keep momentum going to create them.

Yoga chikitsa means "yoga therapy." The main difference between yoga chikitsa and sadhana is that yoga chikitsa is designed to develop a specific skill, like the skill of spaciousness, mindfulness, or deep awareness of self; sadhana applies these skills toward a goal or intention.

Yoga chikitsa becomes your own spiritual yogic prescription to help you find what you picked up this book for in the first place: to connect with your purpose. When you place the smaller, more specific skill practices all together into one collective ritual practice aimed at pursuing a goal — in this case to become more intuitive — this becomes your daily yoga practice, or sadhana. From the yoga chikitsa rituals you have created before, we will now create your intuition rituals. This is your sadhana practice, your own practice, personally created for you by you.

Remember that effective yoga practices are based on what resonates the most with you. While I've introduced several ideas in the course of this book, they don't all need to be part of your regular practices. Start by focusing on the practices that felt easy to understand, that you know you could benefit from, and that you are excited to know more about.

Take time to experiment with various practices and play with different techniques; once you've tested out the available options, then pick your favorites.

Whatever your preconceived ideas of what a yoga practice

looks like, let them go. You can practice yoga in many forms; you don't have to sit on a yoga mat for an hour every day.

I am not a monk. I am a mother, business owner, writer, avid traveler, and friend to many. There was no option for me to run off to a cave to practice yoga, so I started to find ways I could bring yoga into my everyday life, anywhere I felt I could fit it in. Your sadhana is not meant to be another thing on your already overwhelming to-do list, but something that you can do here and there with ease.

Motherhood has taught me to become more adaptable by practicing yoga in baby steps — in rituals. One of my intuition rituals is to take one hundred conscious breaths a day; normally these happen in the shower or while putting my son to bed. These days, I actually practice yoga for less time than I did all those years before, but I do so more consistently, and I feel the benefits all the more because of it. Using this approach, I have manifested some incredible dreams that a few years ago I thought were impossible.

Trust that the baby steps of your rituals are taking you somewhere important, and commit to making them happen as often as you can. The key to a purposeful and meaningful life is surrendering to your intuition. Your intuition rituals will show you how; you just need to listen.

Create Your Intuition Rituals: Vinyasa Krama

Here are a few primary considerations to keep in mind when creating your intuition rituals.

Time. Ask yourself what amount of time you can realistically take in your daily life for practicing your intuition rituals.

Once you get to this point, you will no longer need to practice the other yoga chikitsa rituals in their entirety on a daily basis unless you have extra time or you feel you need more of those elements in your life. The most important thing you can do now is make sure your intuition rituals happen every single day. Begin with a time commitment that is doable, so there is no way you won't achieve it. If you only want to commit to ten minutes a day to start, then do that. If you already have a daily yoga practice, perhaps try making your intuition rituals your daily yoga practice for a while and experiment with how this feels.

Practices. Think about which practices from each of the previous three steps resonate most with you. Now, grab a piece of paper or your journal and make a list of the personalized intuition rituals you intend to create in each of the three categories below. Which of your previous yoga chikitsa practices will be a part of your intuition rituals? Be as specific as you can. Instead of writing "breathing practice," for example, write down exactly which breathing practices you are going to use and for how long.

- **Rituals to create more spaciousness.** What spaciousness practices feel the most powerful to you? Posture yoga? Exercise? Breathing? Relaxation? Hobbies you love?
- **Rituals to create more mindfulness.** What mindfulness practices draw you most strongly? Are there specific breathing practices you can commit to each day? Is there a certain amount of time or a particular number of conscious breaths you can commit to taking?
- **Rituals to create more awareness.** What feeling practices are you most pulled to explore? Yoga nidra?

Chakra meditation? Long Shavasanas with an intention to feel? Relaxation practices? Journaling?

Practice and Adjust

Now that you know how much time you have available and the practices that resonate most strongly with you, include at least one practice from each of the previous steps.

You can always add your yoga chikitsa practices as a weekly or monthly practice, so you keep developing those skills, but in this chapter you want to make sure you create a set of rituals that you do as regularly as possible. For example, it might be difficult to incorporate a yoga nidra meditation on a daily basis, but a weekly or a bimonthly yoga nidra may be doable for you.

Your rituals may need to change over time. If you find that one of the rituals feels difficult for you, spend more time on it. Or perhaps you created your rituals with an overzealous energy but are having difficulty maintaining a daily consistency to your practice. If so, eliminate something. Minimize. On the other hand, perhaps you are ready to add more practices into your rituals after a few weeks. You are the guru; only you can create the perfect rituals for you.

My Intuition Rituals: An Example

To give you a better idea of what your intuition rituals might look like, I will share mine, but remember that in order for intuition rituals to be most effective, they should be created by you and for you.

My personal intuition rituals are designed to take forty-five minutes to one hour each day, separated into morning and afternoon sessions.

I like to number my rituals so I can move through my list every day without forgetting anything. Know that by doing your designated five, ten, or twenty things each day, you are creating the life you want for yourself.

Spaciousness

1. Do at least three to five Sun Salutations daily, more if I feel the desire to add.
2. If time allows, add on postures that I am intuitively drawn to for nurturing the way I want to feel.
3. Do a relaxing heart opening posture on a yoga block for five minutes daily.

Mindfulness

1. Breathe one hundred conscious breaths daily.
2. Perform a breathing practice given to me by yoga teacher O. P. Tiwari that includes *uddiyana bandha* (five rounds), *agni sara* (five rounds), *simha kriya* (five rounds), *Brahma mudra* (five rounds), *nadi shodhana* (five rounds), *bhastrika* (ten rounds), *sitali* (ten rounds), and *ujjayi* (fifteen rounds).

Feeling

1. Do a guided yoga nidra meditation twice weekly.
2. Engage in intuitive journaling as often as possible.
3. Do something I love every single day. Passion leads to purpose.

EXERCISE: *A Dreamer's Journal*

After some time practicing your spaciousness rituals, your mindfulness rituals, and your feeling rituals, experiment with the journaling prompts below to see if you gain clarity on what your passions and your dreams are. These questions may inspire intuitive shooting stars within you. If you feel something special, know it is worth exploring. If you do not feel anything special, just continue practicing your intuition rituals, and the intuitive messages are bound to come as you integrate the necessary skills into your life.

The Who, What, When, Where, and Why of My Dreams

WHO

- Who inspires me?
- Who is living something similar to what I want?
- Who is an example of what I want to become?

WHAT

- What exactly is it that I want to do?
- What am I passionate about?
- What would I like to feel more of in my life?

WHEN

- Imagine manifesting my dreams and contemplate the question: What is delaying me going after my dreams? Write it down.
- As I imagine living my dreams, what do I see that looks different from my current reality?
- How would it feel to be there now?

WHERE

- Where is this idea going to take me?
- Where would I like to see myself in a year?

WHY

- Why do certain people inspire me?
- Why do I want what I am dreaming?
- Why is this so important to me?

The Visualization

If you are clear on your dream, write it out with as much detail and specificity as you can.

Finding Clarity

Finally, complete the following sentences every day.

MY DREAM IS...

- to do _____
- to feel _____
- to be _____
- to have _____

If you lack clarity on what your dream is, then continue practicing your intuition rituals until it becomes clear. When you know what it is you want, how you want to feel, and what your soul is asking you to do, you are then ready to manifest.

7

Unblocking *and* Becoming

If the doors of perception were cleansed,
every thing would appear ... as it is, infinite.

— WILLIAM BLAKE

A few years ago, I took a trip into the Tibetan Autonomous Region of China, the Dalai Lama's homeland before he became a political exile to India. I always dreamed of seeing "the Rooftop of the World," probably more than any other place. The mountains of the region are the tallest on the planet. Its culture and history are rich, and the spiritual beliefs that were born here have spread all over the world.

China had just recently completed a new rail line spanning 2,300 miles, beginning in Beijing and gaining 16,400 feet in altitude at the highest point before pulling into the last stop in Lhasa, Tibet. Lhasa is the capital of the province and was the religious and political center for Tibetan Buddhism until the Chinese forcefully and inhumanely took over the entire country in 1949.

As a tourist to Tibet, I was forced to follow the Chinese authorities' strict rules and guidelines for how I could travel there. I spent weeks in the polluted city of Xining midway along the train journey, organizing all the necessary permits and paperwork required for me to travel through the eerily watched-over province. I had to be escorted at all times by a government-approved guide and hire my own private driver and car to take me anywhere I planned to go. As difficult as the process proved to be, there was no stopping me. I was determined to see this place, to understand its culture, and to spend time with its people.

To my relief, I was appointed a Tibetan guide. Tenzin, who had a warm, sincere demeanor about him, was waiting for me on the train platform as soon as the last horn blew into the station. There weren't many tourists around, so it was easy for him to spot me, the young American girl carrying an oversized backpack with a yoga mat strapped to the side.

From the train station we walked the short distance to our basic little Tibetan homestay in the Barkhor, the old Tibetan part of the city, located around the Jokhang Temple, believed to be the most sacred and important temple in Tibet. *Lhasa* in Tibetan means "place [*sa*] of gods [*lha*]," and it is easy to see why. From our simple room, we could see the towering white presence of the Potala Palace, the fortress that used to be home to the Dalai Lama.

Every time we walked out of our guesthouse, we immediately entered a constant flow of pilgrimaging devotees circling the temple day and night, chanting and praying. Thick-robed Tibetans holding prayer beads were performing full-body prostrations in every direction I looked. The Tibetans' style of full-body prayer involves reaching to the sky with their hands in prayer position, sliding their bodies along the ground to lie flat on the earth, coming back to standing, then taking a step forward and doing it all over again.

Many of these pilgrims had traveled thousands of miles, praying and sliding their bodies along every inch of the way; it was a means of earning merit by burning off past bad karma. These devoted practitioners were filthy, covered in road dirt and grime from head to toe, but to me their spiritual dedication was the most inspiring and purest sight I had ever seen.

The smell of yak butter lamps filled the narrow cobblestone streets, billowing out of the main Jokhang Temple. Inside the walls were covered in black soot from the smoke of candles, incense, and yak butter, always burning, year after year. At this point in my life, I was deeply curious about the different ideologies of religion, especially Buddhism. I walked around with my eyes peeled open, as this was the most confident spiritual display I had ever seen. I needed to know everything: What did the flowing prayer flags mean? And the beads they held in their hands? Why did the people prostrate to the point of pain? Tenzin proved incredibly helpful for explaining the rituals I saw the Tibetans performing throughout the trip and what they signified to the people.

After a week in Lhasa, I threw my dusty backpack in the back of an old white SUV, and Tenzin, our driver, and I began driving across the vast, barren alpine region to the Nepali border. It was already late November by the time we were allowed to begin the journey, and it was getting cold. Along the way we stayed in yak-dung-constructed Tibetan houses where the homeowners would serve us endless cups of yak butter tea as we sat around their simple potbellied stoves to stay warm. I remember shivering through most nights.

We would usually sit in silence, but on occasion the locals from the village would try to share their personal life stories with me in barely comprehensible English. I understood their stories, though, intuitively. They would tell me of a missing cousin or brother, or how they managed to escape to India and meet the Dalai Lama, only to walk back across the snow-covered passes to be with their families again.

It didn't take long to realize just how inhumane the Tibetan people are treated by the ruling Chinese. There is no freedom for the Tibetan people; the Chinese government does not allow them to possess pictures of, speak about, or pray to the Dalai Lama within Chinese-ruled Tibet. The people who shared their stories of escaping to India and returning had risked being shot both ways. If the Chinese believe Tibetans are not honoring their rules, these Tibetans often go missing, never to be seen again.

Many of the stories and explanations they shared with me could have led them to prison or worse, death. I read numerous books on Tibetan Buddhism and the history of the country while traveling there, and most included pictures of the Dalai Lama on the cover or inside. (I now realize I am very lucky not to have been caught with these.) When the Tibetans' eyes would catch a glimpse of His Holiness on the cover of one of those books, they would stop everything they were doing and hold it in their hands, often putting the picture to their forehead and saying a prayer before kindly handing it back.

I always offered these pictures to them to keep, and they always refused. To be caught with a picture of His Holiness would lead to imprisonment, torture, and often death. It simply wasn't worth the risk. They seemed grateful to have touched some sort of physical reminder of him, a rarity indeed there.

Despite the struggles ever present for the Tibetans living in China, I found it incredibly inspiring to see how they very much stayed connected to their religious leader and their spiritual rituals, despite the risks involved. Although they still performed their rituals publicly, most had adapted their spiritual and personal growth practices into more internal practices. I got the feeling that most of the Tibetans I met never lost focus on the spiritual self, staying true to what they believed in their hearts and souls no matter what was happening around them.

The voice of our soul is our truth. Even when everything around us is telling us we are wrong, we must keep listening to this truth. We don't need our senses to validate how we are feeling. We don't even need our external world to agree with how we are feeling. We merely need to stay true to our soul and the guidance it offers us, overcoming any obstacles and struggles that appear along our spiritual path as we align with that truth.

The Tibetans might not be able to vocally and publicly display their full soul truth inside China, but they are very much committed to honoring it within. Many have chosen to escape to neighboring countries like Nepal and Bhutan to pursue their dream of meeting the Dalai Lama or perhaps to receive a Tibetan Buddhist education. It is believed that more than 150,000 Tibetans have made the heroic, long, and incredibly hostile journey across the plateau into safer lands. Their hearts always guide them.

We walk our unique spiritual path by living our life guided by the messages of our soul. Our spiritual purpose for coming here to Earth in this human body is to do just that, to stay focused on what the heart and soul want.

Sometimes we have to leave our home for a new land when

our current life situation isn't conducive to pursuing the visions of our heart and soul. There might be roadblocks that stand in our way. For many of us, the blockages and challenges holding us back from creating a reality of our soul-sent dreams do not come from the external, but from the internal. However, if we compassionately and patiently open ourselves to the obstacles blocking us, we expand ourselves and grow in the areas our heart is yearning toward. This is how we become what our soul is asking from us.

Becoming

When you do finally hear the messages of your soul, you are ready to begin the adventure of birthing a new reality for yourself. The intuition rituals you have created and are hopefully practicing are certain to awaken you to your soul-sent passions and dreams, but pursuing those dreams is where the soul growth and personal development journey really begins. In this sixth stage of yoga, we will learn to act on our intuition by eliminating the false beliefs living within us, realizing that we — rather than the world around us — are the ones holding us back from creating the realities we wish for ourselves.

This step of the process is about seeing one's shadows and flooding light into them, releasing the chains of human suffering and bondage. This is where manifestation starts and the deep transformation happens.

In this stage of yoga, you will learn to unblock many of the walls or protections holding you back from truly getting what you want in this life. We begin to create a new reality for ourselves by transforming, evolving, manifesting, and becoming. I believe the soul sends us our dreams, not because the dreams are so important, but because of the transformation we must undergo in order to achieve them.

The five steps we have covered in the book thus far are crucial to connecting with your intuition and realizing your dreams, but now you will learn to act on those messages by shifting your focus to how you can *become* what you dream. This is where we use the power of looking inside to see what needs to change within us, breaking down those limiting beliefs and misperceptions of who we are and starting to see more truth. This is where we start to feel fearless, strong, confident, and liberated.

In order for us to grow, we must change, and oftentimes it is our greatest difficulties that inspire our greatest awakenings. The sixth step of yoga can be uncomfortable. It demands that you change the way you have always done things so that you can create yourself anew.

The Blockages

Oftentimes, the moment an intuitive dream comes to my awareness, my logical mind immediately reacts by telling me why it isn't possible to achieve. "I would love to study art, but art doesn't make money," I might think, or "I am going to travel the world — when the timing is right." When statements like these arise within you, it means a blockage is keeping you from moving toward your dream.

"But" and "when" statements are what this stage is all about. The excuses that constantly tell you why you can't or won't do something are simply not true. You are a wild, adventurous soul very much on a mission to learn, and the yogis found that sometimes our mind forgets that, especially the logical part of the mind.

Evolutionarily, we have become risk averse. We are meant to fly across oceans like the bar-tailed godwits traveling from Alaska to New Zealand, yet we stay stuck on the shoreline. We are meant to take big adventures in our lives like the caribou who travel 2,000 miles across spongy muskeg and frozen tundra. We are meant to migrate like the monarch butterflies, who experience the death of three generations along their route returning home. We are meant to chase our intuitive dreams because this is how our soul migrates to where it wants to go.

When I began my life as a soul-based entrepreneur just a few years ago, several strong, loud, limiting beliefs were always screaming in my mind. That voice told me, "It seems too difficult," "You are wasting your time," and "You aren't experienced enough to do this." I feared that people would sense my inexperience and call me a fraud.

Humans are brilliant when it comes to self-sabotage. We naturally want to avoid pain and suffering, so we cower away from threats and challenges. We build walls to avoid being seen as vulnerable, to keep the pain out. We choose the path of least resistance so we are guaranteed success and can avoid being viewed as a failure by others. Or we simply procrastinate to the point of never starting, or we start and then quickly give up.

Our soulful dreams are always motivated by passion and heart, not fame and fortune. The happy, soulful part of you who wants to be an artist, a singer, a writer, a business owner, or a dancer may too often underprioritize your passions in favor of the societal virtues of money, stability, security, or success. And while by no means am I encouraging you to give up your job and just wing it, I am asking you to think about what it is that makes your heart beat faster and to prioritize doing *that*, no matter what your inner dialogue or even your outer world is saying against it.

In order to build the successful business I dreamed of, I had to unblock each of my limiting beliefs one by one. I had to find a strength I didn't know I was lacking. I had to become whatever it would take to give birth to the businesswoman, the writer, the mindful mother, the calm and relaxed human I wanted to be.

In order to live a life that felt meaningful, I had to leave Alaska and go on a big walkabout. I left my home, my partner, and my career. All of this took a lot of unblocking. For young Australian Aborigines, a "walkabout" is considered a rite of passage and is believed to focus the wanderer on the motivation of movement rather than the frequency. That's exactly what I was figuring out too, as I wandered.

My trip through Tibet taught me that no matter what difficulties lie ahead of you, you must stay true to your soul's yearning. What are your passions? And what is drawing energy and attention away from you doing what you want with that passion? This is what we are meant to stay focused on above all else.

In this chapter we will learn what the most common blockages are and how to break through them.

Unblocking

Dreams are almost never handed to you. They are made.

I want to encourage you to start telling yourself that you are ready for what your intuition is asking from you. You are powerful enough. This is why your soul chose your specific human body and all the quirks and eccentricities that are you.

You are absolutely perfect for this pursuit. You were made for it. And the only person who is going to help you manifest your dreams is *you*. No one else is as passionate about or inspired to create that reality.

Let's say I want to travel the world; that isn't so far-fetched, is it? Yet I have a terrible phobia of getting sick. If I live in doubt that I can actually do it, I will stay sitting at home, wishing forever to see the Taj Mahal or the Eiffel Tower, longing to see what that experience is like — but never actually going for it.

The sixth step of the yoga process, called *dharana*, is deeply personal. You must get to the roots of yourself and then use the practices to strengthen those roots. B. K. S. Iyengar defines *dharana* as "concentrating wholly on a single point or on a task in which [the practitioner] is completely engrossed." You focus entirely on the seed you are planting and merely pull out all the weeds hindering that seedling's growth. Surprisingly, this step is less about taking action to create the dream and more about clearing all the limiting beliefs and misperceptions blocking you from seeing the clear path to get there.

You do not need to understand exactly why your blockages are present; at first, simply acknowledging what hindrances are alive in you, and seeing them for what they are, is often enough to get you moving forward. When I grab my backpack and walk onto a plane, whatever doubts my mind is raising, I know these are misperceptions living in my anxious mind. I then can find the strength to keep walking forward to do, see, and be exactly what I want.

I promise you, with a little effort every day, the same will happen with your dreams. You will grow closer to them. And as you take a step forward, you might find more blockages on your path. You have to be patient with the process and diligent in continuing to move ahead.

When I started my business, I also found many blockages stubbornly sitting along my path to success. The story of why I was bound to fail started unfolding in my head, one excuse after another, all giving me the same messages: I wasn't good enough, and everyone was sure to see me fall flat on my face. At first I loathed promoting myself as a businesswoman, feeling judged and criticized for every word I wrote. The truth is no one was judging me as harshly as I was judging myself.

I was determined to stay concentrated on my dream to run my own business, but that meant I would need to unblock the fears and insecurities so strongly popping up along the way. One of the things I did was take a course on vulnerability that my friend, breath work teacher, and fellow writer Conni Biesalski was offering. In the course I learned that when we vulnerably share with others our most embarrassing truths, we de-shame them, and naturally they begin to dissolve.

In the first year of entrepreneurship, I realized that I had to stop focusing on my imperfections and redirect my concentration to the business I passionately desired to create. And I did build a successful business for myself, traveling to the world's best surf breaks with groups of like-minded women with an intention to study the soul. I ended up running more than twenty retreats around the world, in Sri Lanka, Bali, France, and Morocco. I did most of it with a baby, too, a process that came with its own set of blockages to overcome!

After I gave birth to my son, at first I was petrified: How would I continue my nomadic career with a child? Once again, I simply found a way to deal with it. My husband and my baby would have to come with me! I have found confidence, courage, and a newfound dedication through my journey. There were things I felt I couldn't do, but when I put my mind to them, I discovered I could. I learned to believe in myself and ignore the logical, cruel, naysaying voice of my belief system. I learned to find my own unique way to do exactly what I wanted to do.

Blockages didn't appear only when I started my business. They rose up when I began to learn how to play an instrument, when I started surfing, when I wrote this book, and even when I moved abroad. This is exactly what the yogis want us to do here — to concentrate on whatever it is that sets your heart on fire. While the five previous steps of yoga together will help you realize your dreams, this step right here, dharana — staying unwaveringly focused on what your soul wants and simply observing and not reacting to all the ways you want to run away from it — is the first key to acting on your soul's messages.

As you deepen your practices, intuitive messages will continue to ping through you over and over again; the speed at which you choose to respond to them is up to you. Thomas Edison made 1,800 attempts before successfully inventing the light bulb. How many times do you think he wanted to give up? His soul kept bringing him back to his invention table time and time again.

Dream manifestation is a journey, an adventure, and an expedition. You will encounter bends and hills along the way that might throw you off course. The key to the sixth step is not to give up; just keep unblocking and rerouting yourself toward truth.

And I must warn you: when you do manifest your dream, people will say to you, "You are so lucky," and a part of you will cringe, because you know that it's really because of the internal shadow work you did that no one else can see. It certainly wasn't luck that got you here, but determined diligence, concentration, and willpower. It is the hard work you put into the sixth stage of yoga, dharana, that allows you to become what you dream.

Life's Five Great Lessons

In yoga, our blockages are called *kleshas*, or afflictions, which stop us from seeing things as they truly are. The kleshas are like veils separating us from our true nature.

In the second book of the Yoga Sutras, the yogis warned us about five common blockages that we will inevitably find through the course of our soul-manifesting lives: *avidya* (misperception), *abhinivesha* (fear), *dvesha* (avoidance), *raga* (craving), and *asmita* (overidentifying with the ego). These are the causes of nearly all of our pain and suffering.

When it comes to manifesting your intuitive dreams, being able to look at your blockages without reacting to them becomes a very important step. When you disconnect from the fear, avoidance, craving, and ego-chasing misperceptions of the mind, you stay grounded on your intuitive path. It becomes easier to see where to go next. You learn to live less from the misguiding direction of your subconscious wounds and more from the fearlessness in your soul.

Iyengar said of the kleshas, "So long as they are not studiously controlled and eradicated, there can be no peace." The kleshas are our life lessons, and the entire eight-step system of yoga was designed to help us see them and rid ourselves of them.

Read over the descriptions of the kleshas that follow. If you feel a strong resonance with one, it is your intuition highlighting the spiritual work ahead for you. Only you know which of the afflictions are creating pain in your life, and only you can stop making decisions from those wounds. Only you know the shadows and trauma within you, and only you can free yourself from them.

When you find a blockage that resonates with you, simply acknowledge it and remind yourself that it is natural for these feelings and thoughts to live within you. They live in all of us. You are finding the speed bumps along the path toward your spiritual maturity; do not mistake them for stop signs. Just observe them for what they are, with patience and compassion. Eventually they will not affect you anymore. When you observe the natural logical and fearful tendencies arising within you but stop living from them, you will start to feel a newfound sense of innate worth, confidence, and unshakable strength. Unblocking is not an easy step by any means, but it is where all the crucial change occurs.

The goal of this step of yoga is to compassionately observe the blockages most affecting your life, see them, know them, even love them, but not live from them. Some may take years or even lifetimes to overcome. This is most certainly a step that takes a lot of deep and hard work; we are changing our subconscious beliefs, after all. In my opinion, this hard work is the reason our soul takes human journeys. Warning: there will be growing pains.

Avidya: Misperceptions

The first blockage explained by the yogis, *avidya*, translates to "misconception, ignorance, misunderstanding, delusion, and incorrect knowledge." Avidya arises when you think you know something, but it isn't actually true. Its opposite is *vidya*, or clarity and truth. The journey to vidya is exactly what the entire human experience is all about. Your dreams, guided by your intuition, are simply taking you on a wild ride so that you can know the truth about yourself and the world around you.

Perhaps this is the first time you have ever considered your dreams in the yogic context we are exploring together here. Because of avidya, misperception, you didn't know about this lens and never perceived life through it.

Many of us walk through life blind to our intuition, never awakening to the guidance and mystical passions it sends through us on a daily basis. As you may have witnessed by now, when you create spaciousness, mindfulness, and conscious awareness of what is happening within you, you may experience an awakening. The yogis gave us the first five steps of yoga — the yamas, niyamas, asana, pranayama, and pratyahara — to help us learn the language of the soul and to find truth for ourselves. Each of the steps offers us a different lens for seeing into ourselves. The eight-step process as a whole is one of self-inquiry, svadhyaya, one of the key virtues for living a spiritual life. Through this process, we are learning to see through a new form of perception, intuition. We are finding what is true for us from our own unique firsthand experience.

Dharana is the bridge that helps us get from ignorance to wisdom, from fake to real, from confused to clear, from stuck to liberated. And through this step of yoga, we learn to discern what is truth, vidya, and what is misperception, avidya. It is a bit like cleaning a dirty window and seeing nature in its clarity just on the other side.

The first klesha creates the field for all the other kleshas to take root. Avidya is simply not knowing any better. All of us humans are here on Earth making mistakes because we simply don't know better. Both Hindus and Buddhists believe that misperceptions come from conditioned imprints adopted throughout our current or past life experiences and affecting our behavior. We make decisions based on fears and ignorance rather than on intuitive soul guidance.

We all have our unique misperceptions, beliefs, wounds, understandings. It's easy to see why we don't always get along, why there are battles and wars in the world and within ourselves. Every single one of us is here on Earth looking for truth; in that way we are all created equal. Luckily for us, as yogis, we have a step-by-step system to follow to find that truth.

This is how the process of soul growth and personal transformation works. This is how we learn. These misbeliefs live deep within us, and we must dig them out to see them. With each wrong turn we take, we get closer to knowing which direction is actually for us. We can quit shaming and scolding ourselves for every misstep of the way, compassionately realize our missteps come from avidya, and continue walking.

Logical versus Illogical Thinking

Logical thinking is one of the greatest misperceptions directly blocking us from our intuition. Although it is most certainly helpful to use logic in many daily situations, it can be a hindrance when it comes to manifesting your intuitive dreams. Logically guiding your life will often be in opposition to intuitively guiding your life. When this clash occurs, a cloud of confusion surrounds everything we do.

Remember that *dharana* translates to "staying completely engrossed in a task." That task is following your soul's guidance.

Stay diligently concentrated on your soul dreams, no matter what they are, no matter how illogical they seem.

Just because something isn't logical doesn't make it impossible; it can often mean you have a misperception about the path that will get you there. You may have to walk away from a situation that feels safe and predictable. The logical path fools us into thinking we are avoiding discomforts and painful experiences, but in actuality we are creating them.

The logical way to get from A to B is to take the big, wide highway. When you live from your intuition, as illogical as it might seem at times, you start to go off-road. As crazy as it feels, you tend to have much less regret. Intuitively feeling your way to a decision is a much more reliable way to ensure your happiness. This is what the yogis have been trying to teach us.

As you sit in silence observing yourself, you will start to notice where misperceptions exist within you. And as you begin seeing these blockages for what they are and not reacting, they will stop blocking you. As you release them, the path becomes much more clear and defined.

When your logical thinking mind chimes in to tell you how "unrealistic" or "risky" your wild idea is, tell the thinking mind that this is how glass ceilings are broken and new innovations come into being. Becoming an explorer, a pioneer, and a leader means leaving the well-trod path. The wilder your dreams feel, oftentimes the less logical the path to actually reach them is.

Now it's time to try a different avenue. Start to observe within yourself what feels logical and what feels intuitive. Trust your intuition, for it is guiding you to your truth. Ask yourself: *What does my soul want? And what is stopping me from moving toward that?*

Abhinivesha: Fear

Fear is the natural response of the nervous system trying to keep you safe and comfortable. And while a healthy dose of fear is indeed necessary for keeping us alive to a wrinkled old age, when the nervous system starts pumping out excessive fear hormones, fear quickly becomes inharmonious to the point of being debilitating. For many of us living in the modern world, especially women, our fears tend to speak to us through a megaphone, sending cruel and self-damning messages like "I can't do that!" or "Not me!"

Fear, *abhinivesha* in Sanskrit, often grows tentacles, like chronic anxiety, digestive issues, and phobias. In the Merriam-Webster dictionary, *phobia* is defined as "an exaggerated usually inexplicable and illogical fear of a particular object, class of objects, or situation." So, for example, if I constantly hold myself back from doing something because of my fear — perhaps a fear of being alone or a fear of rejection and failure — then I know my fear is definitely blocking my path to becoming.

When you ask a group of kindergarten students, "What would you like to be when you grow up?," an enthusiastic outcry of answers often includes responses like "An astronaut," "The president," or "A ballet dancer." Healthy children think without bounds, without fear. Typically excessive fear and worry arise later in our psychological development, as a result of traumas and other painful experiences.

Our innate natural and truthful state is one of fearlessness, vulnerability, and curiosity. We are born believing we can do anything, and ideally, if we stick diligently to the practices of dharana, we can live and die in fearlessness also.

When you learn to acknowledge the ways fear speaks to

you and stop allowing fear to determine your behaviors and actions, naturally you start doing more of what you love, and you genuinely feel better. I have stayed in jobs I hated out of fear that I wouldn't find another that paid as well. I stayed because I feared not being financially secure. I have stayed in romantic partnerships that deep down in my gut I knew were long over. I stayed because I feared the loneliness and heartbreak I might feel. I feared making a mistake and not being able to undo it.

When I finally started walking toward my fears and observing them simply as that, without reaction, peace and wisdom appeared through the clouds. I found myself feeling like I was exactly where I was meant to be.

When excess fear lives within you, your thoughts and feelings bubble out, sending messages of "I am scared," "I fear being hurt," "What if I fail?," "What if it doesn't work out?," or "Everyone will laugh at me." When you hear these messages, observe them for what they are: old memories living in the psyche asking for your attention to heal them.

Answer this: What brings you restlessness and worry (*ud-dhacca-kukkucca*, one of the Buddhist hindrances)? What exactly is holding you back from doing what you want? What is holding you back from feeling the way you want? What are your greatest fears? Write them down now. You will return to them when we start creating your unblocking rituals.

Dvesha: Avoiding Pain and Discomfort

Humans are creatures of habit. We love predictability; there is a comfort in clearly knowing what lies ahead. It is natural to want to stay safe in a bubble where everything is consistent, known, and secure, but if we stay too safe and never take the leap of faith needed to begin our soul's migration, we merely remain complacent, prolonging our fears into a full life lesson.

The third blockage is dvesha, a deep dislike of pain and discomfort. Fear often stems from an avoidance of pain; avoidance is fear's younger brother. There are times in our lives when we fear getting close to people because of the grief we know we will endure when the relationship inevitably ends. Or we fear putting ourselves out in the public eye because of the uncomfortable rejection and public shame we might experience, preferring to avoid it all together.

When we experience rejection, heartache, pain, and grief, we grow the walls of fear thick in a subconscious attempt to avoid feeling these things again. When your defenses are up and you are living in war with your pain, you start to doubt everything that is good and healing for you.

Answer this: Do you avoid feeling pain? If so, how? Are you able to nonjudgmentally observe your pain without reacting to it? Was there a significantly painful event in your past that you are still healing from and that keeps you avoiding certain situations? If you weren't scared of the possible pain it might bring, what would you do?

Doubt

Doubt is a natural distraction for most spiritual seekers. Patanjali refers to doubt as *samsaya*. We usually doubt when we are trying to avoid future pain. Tibetan Buddhists believe that doubt, *vicikiccha* in Pali, is one of the top five hindrances of any pursuit. It can be helpful to ask yourself when you have doubts, *What am I avoiding?*

During my first meditation retreat, I doubted the practices of meditation were working for me, because I feared wasting my time. And rather than patiently floating along the process, simply observing and being with what was naturally happening, I doubted myself into a state of misery through much of the ten days. This doubt made the process painful — which is exactly what all of the blockages will do for us: they create pain.

I have also had many doubts about expanding and trusting in the growth of my business, making myself small out of fear of failure. When fear, doubt, and avoidance take over the psyche, you can easily find yourself living under a safe complacency blanket — which can feel suffocating at times.

In fact, Mother Teresa shared her own own struggle with doubt in a letter to a friend: "I spoke as if my very heart was in love with God — tender, personal love. If you were (there), you would have said, 'What hypocrisy.'"

Patanjali explains in the Yoga Sutras that there are two disruptive forces that take us away from our goals: procrastination, or *pramada* in Sanskrit, and laziness, or *alasya*. These two threads form the fabric of complacency. Indecision is merely procrastination and laziness combined, keeping us small, keeping us sleeping rather than growing. That is precisely what happens when you stay in a situation even though you clearly know that your soul is asking for something different.

This is why we have entire societies whose members doubt the value of their gut instinct or, even more so, deny its existence. You can always ignore the wild epiphanies that come to you, telling yourself, "When I retire I will do that," but the yogis urged us not to wait. It's time to take that complacency blanket off and start facing your fears.

When doubt lives in the psyche, you may think things like "I am not enough," "I am not creative enough," "I am not talented enough," "I am not experienced enough," "I am not ready," and "I will do this when ..." I often hear people dismiss their ability to do something because they doubt their own power. If I had waited until I felt I deserved the title of "expert yogi" before starting my wellness business, I still would be waiting to start. If I had stopped writing because I doubted the worth or perfection of my prose, you wouldn't be reading this book right now.

Create some spaciousness, tap into your breath, and observe yourself as you answer these questions: Do you self-shame? Do certain things trigger insecurity in you? In what area of your life do you feel you aren't enough? How do you doubt yourself? How are you procrastinating on your path to what you want? What are you avoiding so much that it is keeping you from moving toward your dreams?

Raga: Addiction and Attachment

Just as we dislike feeling pain and avoid it in dvesha, we may also experience the other side of this coin: addiction, craving, and being obsessively attached. This is the fourth klesha, *raga*, meaning "attachment to pleasure." In the same way we avoid pain, we often strive for increased pleasure.

Many of us cling to partners and friendships that are no longer helpful for what our soul wants from us, simply because the presence of these people makes us feel worthy. We cling to food or alcohol consumption to make us feel good, because internally we don't. Or we may become addicted to work and external accomplishments because this makes us feel important and purposeful.

When we are hyperfocused on being happy or only feeling bliss, we are avoiding pain. This makes decisions seem much more important than they are. Indecision was one of my greatest struggles when I started my own business. Which logo to choose? How to market myself? What should I write on my website? The list of decisions I needed to make was extensive and exhausting, and by craving results for pleasure I put intense pressure on myself to have all the answers and make the "right" choices.

As you become more intuitive, you are going to need to make more and more decisions, because you are not making the logical, intellectual choice — you are paving a path of your own. Suddenly thousands of doors open up to you, and you have to really feel into the spacious observatory within yourself to know which door your intuition wants you to walk through.

It helps me to remember that the soul guides us much as a GPS does. Even when you make a wrong turn, you will be rerouted in the direction you are meant to be going. So don't focus so much on the results you want to achieve; focus on what feels right in this moment in your body and take action from that. This process is not concerned with your productivity; the purpose is about your transformation.

If you go with your gut, you are guaranteed to get back on the right path. If you aren't sure exactly what your gut is saying, move back through your intuition rituals and spend a little extra time feeling for the answers. Then simply decide. Clarissa Pinkola Estés writes in her book *Women Who Run with the Wolves*, "It is worse to stay where one does not belong at all than to wander about lost for a while and looking for the psychic and soulful kinship one requires." Wander freely, trying new things.

The idea that there is a wrong or right decision is a blockage and a limited way of seeing things. Make your decision and continue on. Simply let happiness float to you, rather than trying to force it. You have much more important things to spend your time and energy on than deciding; you need to keep momentum above all.

I have a personal motto that I tell myself when I struggle to make a decision: "If I can't decide, it probably doesn't matter."

Answer this: Do you use relationships, productivity, success, or substances to make you feel better? What are you clinging to in order to make yourself feel good? What do you desperately yearn for in your life, and why? Do you become indecisive because you are searching for one possible outcome? Once you are clear on that, you can start to see how your addictions and cravings bring you misery and suffering, and indecision jumps in to stumble you up.

Asmita: Ego Chasing

As our fears, cravings, and aversions are illuminated, so too will be the ways we tend to chase the ego — the ways we go after fame and fortune to prove our worthiness. *Asmita*, being ego driven, is the fifth blockage listed by the yogis. When we are chasing a dream in order to make ourselves feel more beautiful or successful, because we do not feel these emotions innately within ourselves, this is a form of ego chasing. This is a way we try to make ourselves feel worthy, but our worth never comes from this.

When we are chasing dreams for superficial reasons, it never leads to the worth, purpose, and contentment our dreams are meant to lead us to. The greatest thing we can do to begin to feel worthy is to understand that we are all souls on our soul journey. Only when you understand how sacred you are — even without the money, appearance, intellect, and success society says you're supposed to have — can you truly stop chasing dreams from a place of ego and start chasing them from your soul purpose.

When you understand that you are here to feel for your intuition and act on it, all the superficial tactics for proving worthiness start to fall away. You don't need the fancy car, the gold medal, the six-figure income, the storybook partner to feel you are important and have a purpose. You don't need to be your mind's picture of perfect. You simply can be what you feel, what you are learning, your true and vulnerable self.

Don't get me wrong: external praises, fame, and fortune may still appear in one's life, but let them appear without chasing them. The Dalai Lama lives with an abundance of fame and wealth, but his intention is not to possess these things. He is simply living his truth, guided by what his heart tells him to do, and fame and wealth have naturally manifested around him. You will see the same happen for you.

The Buddhists teach that sensory desire, *kamacchanda* in Pali, is one of the ways we pull ourselves out of our inner world and back into the superficial. It is one of the five Buddhist hindrances. Upon ordination, Buddhist monks and nuns are instructed to immediately discard their lay clothes, sleep on a simple mattress low to the floor, and eat only what has been donated. When you return to minimalism and simplicity, the ego cravings become easier to unblock. The problem with ego-fueled materialism is that you are attached to external things as a means of feeling more secure and worthy. Ultimately the soul wants you to feel worthy and secure in yourself simply for being a growing soul. It is easier to learn to do that without external things.

If you realize at some point you have been chasing something because it will help you feel more worthy, more important, more prestigious, or more valuable, know that this is an ego-sent dream, not your soul's path and purpose but rather an obstacle to it. Not being wasteful is also one of the yamas, the rules the yogis mentioned to us and which we discussed in chapter 2: *aparigraha*, meaning "to simplify or minimize."

In India, at the end of a Hindu's life, it is common practice to give up all his or her material possessions and spend the final days as a homeless renunciant, shedding the ego fully before being forced to shed the human body as well. Another common tradition in India is for women to shave their heads, dispelling the egoistic veil of vanity and beauty.

The goal is always to return home to your soul, to your truth, to your self.

I must be honest with you: the yoga strategy I am teaching you can be used to manifest ego dreams, like money and fame, in the same way it can be used to manifest your soulful ones. You sometimes do not know until after your manifestation comes true that it wouldn't bring you the feelings and embodiment you were after; then it becomes clear it was an ego dream. Another way these manifestations can play out is that you become incredibly powerful and skilled in the process, developing siddhis and superpowers, which can fuel the ego and turn pride into arrogance.

That's why I want to be clear with you: Your dream isn't the ultimate goal. It's merely a tool for soul growth through the eight-step yoga process.

Ask yourself: What stories do you want to have associated with your name? What do you do just to feel more purposeful and important? Could you give up these things, or are you clinging to them? Get to the heart of why you do everything you do. When you do, suddenly the ego is shed, and the soul light shining from within you can be seen by all around.

The Unblocking Practices

The traditional yoga way to unblock includes gratitude practices, affirmations, visualizations, and deep meditations. Luckily for us, in our modern times, we have additional endless unblocking support available to us. A few contemporary practices for helping you unblock might include life coaching, personal development courses, cognitive behavioral therapy, and neurolinguistic programming.

Every dream must come with a strong intention and commitment; otherwise, complacency and procrastination take over. In Sanskrit, this noncommitment or absence of vows or resolutions is called *avirati*. Avirati is when we know we want to manifest a dream but are unsure exactly how to get there, so we never take any action. This is why your rituals are so important; you commit to making them happen every day, no matter what.

Now you are committing to seeing the reality of why you do things and why you don't, thus growing ever closer to your innate true nature.

Relaxation

Our limiting beliefs live in our subconscious mind. Relaxation is a good place to start to loosen the misperceptions living within you and free yourself from them. Through deep, intentional relaxation, you move into the realm where your blockages live.

By minimizing stress and staying relaxed through the journey, simply observing the blockages as they arise and pass away, you keep the channel of intuitive communication open. From this calm place, you find that your blockage ceases to exist anymore and you can easily get back on track.

Relaxation is a skill you get better at with practice. As we've discussed earlier, relaxation techniques include mindful meditations, body scanning, tai chi, qigong, massage, and Reiki; there's also float therapy, restorative yoga, and progressive relaxation techniques. Anything that relaxes you works. If there is an activity that you feel keeps you open and soft, do it on a regular basis.

You may find that some blockages will diminish on their own through relaxation, like fear-based anxiety and indecision, while other blockages might become clearer. The following unblocking practices might come in handy for the latter.

Affirmations

Affirmations are a yoga technique offered by Patanjali himself. Yoga Sutra 2:33 states, "Upon being harassed by negative thoughts, one should cultivate counteracting thoughts." Tell yourself whatever it is that you need to believe when the mind tells you you shouldn't.

Affirmations help you manifest the change you desire in your life by rewiring the neurological connections of your subconscious mind. Essentially, when you use affirmations, you are encouraging your mind to perceive things about yourself and the world by telling it how to think differently. Affirmations can be helpful for unblocking all the kleshas: misperception, fear, aversion, craving, and ego desiring.

When it comes to self-doubt, insecurity, fear, procrastination, and general weakness, affirmations are especially powerful. With consistent repetition, your mind begins to believe that the affirmation is a fact, and your brain starts to function as if it is.

Using affirmations is easy and takes very little time. Affirmations are simply statements, always in the present tense, that begin with "I am." It is best to keep your affirmations positive and in the now. For example, instead of saying, "I no longer need cigarettes," you would tell yourself, "I am completely free from addiction." Make your affirmations something you truly want to feel and embody, and then state them as a fact with conviction. Repeat them as often as possible.

I saw firsthand the power of "I am" statements when I was a ski instructor in Alaska. Whenever I met a student who began a lesson by saying, "I am going to the top of the mountain," he or she nearly always did just that. Conversely, students who said, "I do not want to fall," unfortunately seemed to fall a lot. Affirmations work by retraining the brain toward what to focus on — so when you state an affirmation as a negative, you are retraining the brain to focus on that. It's important to concentrate on what you want, not what you are avoiding.

To get you started, let me offer you my ten favorite affirmations: I am happy. I am healthy. I am confident. I am worthy. I am creative. I am loving. I am kind. I am compassionate. I am peaceful. I am a human living my soul's purpose.

If you have one affirmation that you would like to work on, write it on a piece of paper and place it on your bathroom mirror, on your fridge, or in your wallet. Every time you see the words or think about them, say them a few times to yourself.

And then watch what happens. Your brain, mind, body, and life start to become precisely that.

Yoga Nidra

Yoga nidra — the neurological practice you learned in chapter 5 — is a form of neurolinguistic programming that has been used since long before that scientific term ever existed. In yoga nidra meditation, relaxation meets affirmation. In Sanskrit, *nidra* translates to "sleep"; entering this state allows us to work in the subconscious belief layer of our consciousness. Yoga nidra can be a powerful tool for letting go of past trauma, stress, and other painful experiences stored in your subconscious, freeing up that space.

Every yoga nidra practice begins with an affirmative intention, the sankalpa we discussed earlier. This intention sinks into the subconscious as you relax, moving deep into your belief layer. The *vijnanamaya kosha* — the deep subconscious layer of intellect, thoughts, and beliefs — is where your blockages live. By moving your affirmations into this layer, you show your brain exactly how you would like it to think and act.

Visualizations

Visualizations are muscle memory practices for your brain. As dreamers, we use visualizations to prepare our brain for our big moment of manifestation. In the same way an athlete practices for a big game, visualizations help us prepare for the at times arduous journey of dream chasing.

Visualization is a well-developed method of performance

improvement, a fact supported by substantial scientific evidence, and it is used by successful people across a range of fields. As we visualize in the mind what we want to become, new neural pathways are created in the brain, training it to become alert to the people, resources, circumstances, and opportunities that will actually make the visualization a reality.

One of my favorite visualization stories comes from the life of Natan Sharansky. Sharansky was an Israeli Jew who spent nine years in prison in the USSR after he was accused of spying for the United States. While in solitary confinement, he played himself in mental chess.

Sharansky had been a passionate chess player since he was a child, but in those nine years in prison, he never actually had the opportunity to play anyone besides himself. Remarkably, upon his release in 1996, Sharansky beat world-champion chess player Garry Kasparov. Some would call this a miracle, but more so it is proof of the power of the visualization practices.

Visualization works best when you imagine yourself in the state of having manifested your goals. Imagine the excitement, satisfaction, and thrill you will experience when you reach your goals. Visualize your facial expressions and imagine how you will likely feel in that moment. What does manifestation actually feel like? Use visualization practices to get as detailed as you possibly can so that your brain will be well prepared for your moment of manifestation whenever it arises.

Gratitude

Another tool for using the brain's natural neuroplasticity (its ability to retrain) is gratitude. By spending a few minutes a day listing the reasons you are grateful, you are rewiring your brain to focus on the positive rather than the negative. This is how you train the brain to see opportunities rather than resistances to your dreams. You learn to fear less and trust more.

In psychology it is well-known that neurons that consistently fire together will wire together. In other words, a daily ritual of gratitude will change the way you perceive things permanently. You will start noticing more things you enjoy and do them more often. You will focus on the opportunities already in your life and encourage more to float toward you. The brownie point of gratitude practice is that it is sure to make you happier, too.

In fact, the antidepressant medications Prozac and Wellbutrin help produce the biochemical reaction that gratitude creates naturally. Wellbutrin boosts dopamine, and Prozac boosts serotonin; gratitude boosts both. Feeling gratitude is a scientifically proven practice for increasing happiness, by naturally creating these hormones within you. More happiness leads to a more relaxed life, and a relaxed life means a more intuitive, soulful life.

To start a gratitude practice, every day list at least five things that you are grateful for or that make you happy. Then increase it to ten. You can list the same things over and over again, but make sure you stop at some point each day and take note of what you love about your life. I believe gratitude is the key to seeing pathways for manifesting your dream that you might not have noticed before. Oprah has said, "I live in the space of thankfulness — and for that, I have been rewarded a million times over. I started out giving thanks for small things, and the more thankful I became, the more my bounty increased. That's because — for sure — what you focus on expands. When you focus on the goodness in life, you create more of it."

Postures for Power

Traditionally, the ancient yogis of India were considered healers and teachers. Their followers and students would come to them in the hopes of finding relief and healing for anything and everything. When someone complained of a scattered mind and lack of concentration, the yoga gurus might prescribe mindful breath work and/or meditation. If a student was struggling with procrastination and laziness, the yoga teacher might recommend inversions and more dynamic yoga postures to build up to.

You can use particular postures for unblocking because postures help you embody specific feelings. When your body feels tired, use a relaxation posture like Child's Pose or Shavasana. When you are feeling insecure, practice inversion postures, which bring the heart above the head, for strength and confidence. When you are grieving, practice open-heart postures to help you move through and release emotions stuck in the lungs and heart area. If you are overwhelmed with fear, practice learning to trust yourself with balancing poses like Crow.

Flexibility practices, where you hold poses for up to three minutes, teach you patience. Chest openers and backbends expose your heart and help you become more vulnerable. Arm balances create strength and confidence. Twists develop your ability to digest difficult situations as you breathe through uncomfortable, restricting circumstances. You can manifest any feeling by making a ritual of the postures that guide you to feel that way.

I call this style of practice "intuitive yoga" — the use of yoga postures to enhance your life in the specific ways you need. Postures are not to be checked off as you accomplish them, but to be held for longer and longer as you become more comfortable with them. As your life changes, your intuition will guide you to different intentions, postures, and practices. Let your postures change as your life does.

To use physical yoga postures as a method for manifesting a particular feeling within yourself, you must first ask yourself these questions:

- How was I feeling before coming to the yoga mat?
- What would I love to feel more of in my life right now?
- Would I like a deep relaxation? More flexibility? The feeling of freedom? More confidence? More grounding? More focus?
- What postures can make me feel more of this in my life?

I believe that by giving your intuition superiority over decisions and control for creating your own asana (posture) practice, you become your own guru. The asanas your intuition is leading you to do could be in preparation for the big dream. For example, in the years prior to starting my own business, I spent a lot of time practicing arm balances and inversions. Now, I realize that my intuition was pushing me toward these strength-building postures in preparation for the big leap of faith I was about to take.

One of my favorite books for designing an intuitive yoga practice is not specifically a yoga book, but rather a healing book: Louise Hay's *Heal Your Body*. In her brilliant and well-loved bestseller, Hay explains how emotions manifest as pain and illnesses within our physical bodies. Furthermore, she says, each body part represents something specific in the bigger picture of our lives. Hay's insights on what the different areas of the body represent can provide a helpful framework for deciding what to focus on in your practices.

Meditative Breathing

Meditative breathing is the greatest tool for releasing all blockages and making the needed space for creating something new. Meditative breathing is helpful for letting go of what isn't serving you, even if you're not yet sure what that is. Through mindfulness breathing practices, you can learn to surrender control of the things you cannot change and grab the reins of the things you can.

Buddhists believe meditative breathing reprograms the mind by clearing out our samskaras, or unconscious habitual tendencies. As the samskaras vanish from your life, their side effects — anger, depression, anxiety, addictions, intense fear, and attention deficiencies — reduce and may even eventually dissolve completely. As they disappear, the healthiest and happiest part of you gains room to grow.

I feel that meditation has been the greatest cure for all of my mental struggles, especially anxiety. The more I develop my mindfulness, the less I worry, feel nervous, or become jealous. I have increased my clarity. As I learned to redirect my attention to the meditative breath, I have come to live much more in the present moment and have dissolved the antiquated beliefs that were keeping me feeling stuck.

Mentors and Teachers

When I began my business, I tried to do everything myself in an effort to save as much money as possible. I wrote blog posts and magazine articles. I set up photo shoots and turned those photos into advertisements. I networked with anyone and everyone. I organized the retreats, the yoga schedule, the food menu, transportation, temple visits, surf lessons, and more. I didn't know what I needed to do to make my business work, so I did all of it.

Quickly, burnout set in, and I realized I couldn't do it all. Do yourself a favor and accept the support of people in your life in the areas where you most need it! The greatest thing you can do when you are going after something big is to open yourself up to support.

Many modern-day spiritual teachers, including some I haven't met personally, have supported me on my journey to manifestation. One of my greatest inspirations, Eckhart Tolle, has influenced millions of people around the world regarding the importance of mindfulness. In his book *The Power of Now*, he offers his readers a simple and approachable explanation of presence and mindfulness.

Brené Brown's work on the subject of vulnerability has taught me how to live more truthfully and vulnerably. I have turned to her TED Talk *The Power of Vulnerability* many times in moments when I was struggling to take a big leap of faith. Abraham-Hicks's explanation of the law of attraction helped me understand the power of personal and universal magnetization. Esther Hicks's *The Law of Attraction* changed the way I word my affirmations. Now, I try never to ask for something in terms of what I *don't* want, but instead keep the focus on what I *do* want.

When conducting my own experiments from Pam Grout's *E-Squared: Nine Do-It-Yourself Energy Experiments That Prove Your Thoughts Create Your Reality*, I gained confidence in the power of my own mind to bring anything I wanted into my life. In her book, Grout instructs her readers to ask for a clear, unmistakable sign, something that cannot be written off as co-incidence, within a time limit of forty-eight hours, to prove to them that the power of the mind can very much exist in a field of infinite potentiality when we choose it this way.

I remember once sitting on the side of a stunning bay in Morocco and asking for some sort of proof that an energy field existed. An hour later, I went out in the water and had the best surf of my life, catching wave after wave for insanely long dis-tances. When I returned back to the villa where I was staying, many people told me it seemed like I was the only one out in the water; I seemed to be "in the zone." I took that as my sign. Then, the more I came to believe in the power of an intentional mind, the more magical results I experienced.

Mentors and teachers can be found not only in the books you read, but in your parents, your yoga teachers, your life coaches, your friends, or a stranger in the waiting queue at the bank. Anyone who is offering you guidance and support can help you unblock your blockages. These are the people I con-sider soul mates, as they are here to help you connect with your soul. And remember that inspiration is one of the greatest ways to unblock. Find someone who inspires you and use them as an example — a mentor — to continue your unblocking process.

A Supportive Community

Sangha is a Sanskrit word meaning "company" or "community." In Buddhism, a sangha consists of the monks, the temples, and the people you meet there. Finding your personal sangha (even if it isn't religious), your community of like-minded friends, will help you stay motivated. When you tell someone your dream and they get super excited about it with you, this encourages you to get up and make it happen.

When I began running my yoga retreats, I intentionally marketed to people I called "intuitive dreamers," because I wanted to make sure I was gathering the like-minded community of my dreams. Around the fifth retreat, I realized there was an element to each of my gatherings that left me feeling deeply understood. I felt healed and inspired after spending a week with these women, who just days before had been strangers. My retreats were more than a business venture; through them, I was empowered. I felt that I finally fit in.

EXERCISE: *Journaling for Unblocking*

This journaling exercise will help you clarify what your dreams are. Then you will be ready to create your unblocking rituals to bring these dreams closer to reality.

Acknowledge What You Want

If you don't know what you want, how are you ever going to get it? In this exercise, let's try to get clear on what it is you really want. Intuitively answer the questions that follow in your journal. You could ask one question before your daily intuition rituals practice and see if you have gained a clear answer afterward. The more specific you are about what your dream is, the easier it will be for you to manifest it.

WHAT IS YOUR DREAM?

Ask yourself: *What is my dream? Do I feel a magnetization to do something special? Is there a wild and crazy idea that keeps popping up in my mind? Do I have epiphanies? What gets me excited about the future?*

WHAT ARE YOUR PASSIONS?

Ask yourself: *What motivates me? What excites me? What am I most passionate about?* Curiosity, inspiration, and passion are signs that point to what our heart is magnetized toward.

WHAT PEOPLE INSPIRE YOU?

Ask yourself: *Who inspires me? And why are they inspiring to me? What is it that these people are doing that makes them resonate with me?* Look around you and make a list of people who make you feel either inspired or envious or both. When you feel envious, it means there is something about this person that you want but don't yet have. Find out what you believe you are lacking and start growing that within yourself. What do all these inspiring people you listed have in common? Could that be something you want for yourself?

Acknowledge Your Blockages

Once you have clearly stated your dreams in your mind, you need to figure out how you are self-sabotaging your manifestations. Answer this: My dream is _____, but I feel I can't manifest it because _____. Ask yourself: *What is stopping me from taking that big leap of faith? Is fear holding me back? Am I scared of what others will think of me? Do I feel unworthy to manifest this dream? Do I feel I deserve it? Why am I not living my dream now?*

When you see a blockage being communicated in your answers to these questions, consider all the different blockages we discussed and see if you can label the blockage in your own specific situation. Each time you notice blockages in your thoughts, take notes. In the same way that you pull lint from a sweater, start plucking the blockages away, one at a time.

Create Your Unblocking Rituals: Vinyasa Krama

Learning to face your discomforts is a critical step you must take in order to make it all the way down the road to success. Use the unblocking techniques earlier in this chapter to begin changing your mindset. Follow the steps below to help you create your rituals for unblocking the thoughts that stand in your way.

Permission. If your soul was your guide, where would it be leading you? Are you giving yourself permission to fully accept this dream or intention? How can you fully give yourself permission to act on your intuition? Can you make a commitment to yourself right now that you want to start living a more soulful life and are going to dedicate yourself to the practices that will help you do just that?

Visualization. What is your dream? Now, visualize it in as much detail as you can. What does living your dream look like and feel like for you?

Personal unblocking. Decide which blockage resonates most strongly for you right now. That is the immediate blockage you will deal with. Read through the list below and find an unblocking practice you can use to heal it.

- **Unblock self-doubt** by making a list of all the things you doubt about yourself. Once that list is complete, make another list of all the things you are proud of. Now, create an affirmation that is the opposite of your

self-doubt. For example, if you doubt your prepared-
ness for new tasks, repeat to yourself, "I am ready. I am
capable."

- **Unblock a lack of confidence** by listing all the things
  that make you unique and special. Create an affirmation that affirms the opposite of your lack of confidence — for example: "I am worthy. I am talented. I
  am smart."

- **Unblock fear** by visualizing and journaling about how
  you actually see your dream manifesting. Fear is purely
  anxiety about the unknown, so try to plan out the path
  ahead in a way that makes you feel calmer about it.
  Create an affirmation that cuts through your fear and
  brings you peace, such as "I am healthy and happy. I
  am relaxed and ready." Make sure to add a daily relaxation and a mindfulness practice to your rituals to
  calm the nervous system down.

- **Unblock procrastination and distractions** by visualizing what your dream will look like when fully manifested. Build the rituals to support your plan and then
  diligently practice them! Create an affirmation that
  makes you feel ready and centered. Use the mantra
  "There is no time like the present!" to keep yourself in
  the moment.

- **Unblock indecision** by practicing your intuition rituals
  more frequently. This will enable you to make clearer
  decisions. Use the mantra "If I cannot decide, it does not
  matter." Know that if you make the wrong decision, it's
  merely a step on the way to finding the right one.

- **Unblock giving up** by looking within to find out
  what is making you want to give up and focusing your

energies there. Use introspection for as long as you
need to in order to discover why you want to give up.
Oftentimes the dream might still be alive in our heart,
but we don't want to live with stress or worry; if that's
the case, perhaps try to let the process be easy. What
about your current approach isn't working for you,
and how can you change it to better suit you?

- **Unblock overactive logical thinking** by giving yourself permission to follow your intuition, which is illogical — or, as I like to call it, magical.

8

Belief *and* Trust

The most beautiful and profound emotion we can experience
is the sensation of the mystical. It is at the root of all true science.
That deeply emotional conviction of the presence
of a superior reasoning power, which is revealed in the
incomprehensible universe, is my idea of God.

— ALBERT EINSTEIN

A few weeks after my family arrived in Sri Lanka to begin creating our dream life, my husband told me he was leaving me. In the blink of an eye I found myself alone in a foreign country with no community, a single mother, emotionally devastated. I was in the middle of renovating a home for all of us to live in and building a yoga *shala* for my students to gather and study in. While I was growing closer to my dreams, so close I could actually touch them, I suddenly lost my way.

Instantly, my world fell apart. My heart shattered into a million pieces. I was left feeling utterly alone and absolutely broken. I was brought to my knees. Unsure where to look for hope, I started staring at the stars, just as I had all those years earlier in Alaska.

But this time, when I looked at the stars, I learned to connect with the universe as the ultimate commander of my life's journey. I put my hands in the air and stayed that way for nearly a year — 2020, the great year of learning how to surrender for so many of us.

One night, soon after my husband told me he didn't love me, I impulsively bought a plane ticket with tears streaming down my face. I was going to Varanasi, India, a place I believe to be the holiest city in all of India, during the annual Shiva festival. The Maha Shivaratri festival is a spiritual pilgrimage that takes place along the banks of the Ganga River in honor of the Hindu Lord Shiva, the god of transformation. Spiritual seekers come from all over the world for the celebrations.

It has always been hard for me to take a trip away from my son, especially to another country, much less in the midst of family turmoil, but I strongly felt I needed to do this for myself. Luckily my husband agreed to take care of our son, and so off I went on my own, in search of something, again. This time I was looking for some sort of mystical power in hopes that it could take my suffering away and make my husband love me again. I was praying for a miracle.

The moment I arrived in the lobby of my hotel, I met a young Brazilian woman, Natasha, who was also traveling around India alone. We quickly became spiritual companions for the week.

During the seven days of the colorful and deeply moving spiritual festival, we wandered in and out of temples and stayed up all night listening to meditative Hindustani Dhrupad, a form of music that is believed to connect you to your consciousness. I bowed my head to exotic-looking gods and placed my hands at their feet. I asked them to offer me some sort of reprieve from my pain. At first I didn't quite know why or how to pray to the many four-armed, ten-headed elephant gods abundantly scattered around the city; I just started to do it. I touched the feet of the deity statues and then placed my hands on my heart and third eye, just as I saw the locals doing. I poured milk and water over the phallic Shiva lingams whenever we came across them in our wanderings. I sat beside the firepits with the priests and listened to them chanting ancient mantras while ringing bells and banging on drums. Eventually, I started to feel the energetic powers of Varanasi's temples and the mystical energies they held.

One day, while walking along the sacred Ganga River, Natasha and I passed a humble little Kali temple hidden beneath a set of ancient stone stairs. I felt an incredible magnetic urge to go inside and pray to the goddess. With a blood-red tongue hanging out of her mouth and an eerie necklace made of skulls dangling from her neck, the Goddess Kali is a fierce, mean-looking deity who is believed to destroy the evil darkness within us so we can transform it into good. She is often associated with childbirth, as it is the pain and discomfort of childbirth that leads to our greatest love, our children. Kali is our reminder that the path isn't always easy, but she is the key to transforming. She embodies all the strength we need through life's process of becoming.

A few Kali devotees dressed all in black sat on the entry steps smoking cigarettes. They welcomed us inside. The temple walls were painted black, giving the holy shrine a dark energy. Next to the deity's statue sat a middle-aged woman with a hardened face full of wrinkles; my intuition told me she was filled with grief and anger. As I kneeled down beside her, my entire body was overwhelmed with sadness. I wondered if her child had been killed or had taken his or her own life.

Feeling uncomfortable in the heaviness of Kali's home, Natasha and I bowed down, touched the feet of the goddess, and quickly left. It felt like something I needed to do at that exact moment. Something about that woman's sadness made me feel my own misery so clearly. Perhaps it was my own grief and anger I got in touch with in that temple.

I have no doubt that my intuition was guiding my wanderings that day. Immediately after walking out of the Kali temple, Natasha told me she felt a strong urge to go right away to the main Shiva temple a little further down the river. Now it was her intuition guiding us.

Inside the Shiva temple, the energy was warm, comforting, and uplifting, unlike the heavy energy in the Kali temple. As I sat there watching the fire flickering while reciting prayers to Shiva, I sensed a spiritual healing balm being placed right on the open wound that Kali had just opened within me. It felt like a clearing, an opening, and a release.

When we left the temple, a young Brahman priest came running after us demanding to smear devotional ash on our foreheads. Hindus perform this devotional ritual to help the powers of Shiva to enter us so we can continue transforming and growing through our darkness and sadness. Moments later, with three thick white lines spread along the entirety of our foreheads and a big red dot carefully placed on our third eyes, I realized how powerful the art of prayer is — not because of the decorations on my face, but because of the energy shifts, awareness, and acceptance it was offering me. The experience gave me hope at a time when inspiration and motivation seemed to have vanished completely from my life.

When we left the Shiva temple that day, I felt a sort of re-birth. All the praying I had spent the week doing was not in blind faith anymore; in this moment I felt the energy of these temples and deities, what the Hindus call shakti, moving within me. I felt alive. I felt spiritual. I finally felt okay. Perhaps I had even learned to embody the shakti of the gods and goddesses I was spending so much time praying to.

Each of the deities of the Hindu religion holds its own specific energies and miraculous superpowers; that is why, during certain times in our lives, we might spend more time at one temple honoring one particular deity. Similarly, in Hinduism at different times you might change the way you pray, whom you pray to, and the reasons for which you are praying. By first entering the Kali temple, which awakened all of the pain and emotional darkness living within me, and then entering the Shiva temple and feeling that pain transform into growth and power, I understood how each god can be used to support us in different stages of our process.

When you are on your knees sobbing on the bathroom floor, this is when you might start to reach for a miracle. It was the painful death of my college boyfriend that first opened my eyes to yoga as a spiritual practice, and it was when my life seemed to fall apart emotionally that I started to experiment with the power of prayer. Here I was, twenty years after the first event, on the same search for answers. These have been the most ego-shattering and soul-connecting experiences of my life; they have also been the most painful. While I might have cried a lot during the long and lonely journey that 2020 would take me on, I also learned the most about myself through it.

Death and devastation have continuously guided me back to the mystical, the occult, and the unknown. The seventh step of yoga teaches us to surrender to the bigger picture of our existence, even if we might not yet know exactly what that looks like. We learn that we are not in control of many aspects in our lives, such as other people's actions or the timing of events. Prayer is a way for us to feel connected to whatever powers ultimately *are* in our control.

The seventh stage of yoga, called *dhyana* in Sanskrit, is integration and absorption. Dhyana is a step dedicated to believing in yourself and trusting the world around you. This is where you take a leap from the nest and the wind catches you. This is how you learn to soar, whether you feel your life is falling apart or not.

After a soul-shaking week in Varanasi of chanting, offering incense to the gods, and praying and meditating for countless hours, I returned back home to my problem reality in Sri Lanka with a new passion and curiosity to learn more about the energy of shakti. To my surprise, the universe began showering more gifts on me than ever before. Miracles entered my life in the form of serendipitous encouragements. Not with my husband, but with seemingly everything else.

While in India, I felt a strong intuitive desire to learn to play the sitar, one of the Hindustani instruments I meditated with during the all-night musical performances of the festival. Now, back at home, with no idea of how to learn the complex instrument, at the brink of the world locking down because of the pandemic virus Covid-19, a young Indian woman approached me through social media and asked if I would like to take online lessons from her. It felt like a sign — like magic. How could I say no?

During our first class together, my newfound sitar teacher, Nandita, taught me a prayer to the Hindu goddess of learning, literature, music, and the arts, Saraswati. "Saraswati evokes learning within us," she told me. I then shared with her that I was hoping to find a literary agent and publisher for a book I had written over the past few years. I asked her if Saraswati was the best deity for me to pray to for support in this dream. "Saraswati, the goddess of literature as well as music, is most certainly the goddess for you," Nandita responded. "Pray to her as often as you can." So I did.

Since we were both now in strict home lockdowns in our respective countries, we decided to have sitar lessons every single day. We never talked about what was happening in my personal life; she simply taught me to play, and she taught me to pray.

Some days all I wanted to do was cry and watch cartoons with my son, Kona, on the couch, but when I showed up to class, I was forced to turn my emotional voice down and listen to the subtle sounds of the sitar with all the concentration I could muster. Nandita gave me the discipline and routine I needed when my life and the world seemed to be falling into chaos. She taught me the prayers I needed to know. She gave me the wisdom of an instrument and taught me how to meditate with it, which inspired and motivated me to meditate more, just when I most desperately needed to.

In the same way that the little girl I saw living at the orphanage in Zambia danced through her days, I too would learn to use music to bring joy into my days, despite the desperation I was so painfully feeling inside. One of my uncles, who has been playing music since he returned home as a Vietnam veteran, once told me, "Music fills the void." And so for me, in this time of my life, it has.

For the first time in my life, I could see creativity and art as pure expressions of my inner process. I realized just how healing it is to simply strum the sitar, sing, write, paint, and otherwise create. The more I passionately created, the more free I felt from the strong emotions sitting so heavily inside of me. Art, music, and writing became intuitively guided practices constantly connecting me with my soul.

Now, when I play the sitar, I feel the vibrations of the music moving through the immense spaciousness within me — a big, open emptiness of the grief left inside me. When I feel for the music moving through me, it is a reminder that I am still alive. I travel into the cellular parts of myself, mindfully engaging in the sounds of the music and how they dance in my body. This subtle way of meditating has shown me the deepest level of consciousness I have ever known. I can only speculate that this must be the place Einstein would passionately take himself with his beloved violin when his magnificent discoveries came to him.

When I was first learning to play from Nandita, I started to see the clouds parting, and life started to feel loving again. Many good things were happening — enough, in fact, to give me a sense that the universe was slapping me in the face while saying, "We are supporting you, woman! Keep doing your art and keep asking for what you want!" I began to understand that the space my husband chose to create between us was an invitation for us to start over with a new dynamic, free from the relational habits that for years were unconsciously running the show. It was an invitation for me to be open, patient, and compassionate with the process of letting our relationship become whatever it wanted to be, authentically. I learned to be authentically me. He learned to be authentically him. If we could be together in peace, that was great. And if not, I would learn to be okay with that also.

I found a new confidence and sense of worthiness developing within me as a result of the devotional rituals I had learned on that trip to India, so I kept diving deeper and deeper into the occult practices of yoga. You can be sure that I was soon singing my Saraswati mantra a little louder and with a little more care than before. I sang it like I really meant it.

For the next few months, I sat alone in my little jungle house in Sri Lanka, studying Vedic astrology, meditating with mantras to the sounds of my sitar, and learning about each of the different powers one can invoke through all the many gods.

While you most certainly are in control of 75 percent of what happens in your life, the other 25 percent is controlled by the universe, God, or whatever bigger power you believe in. This step of dhyana teaches us how to trust in the other 25 percent. In her book *The Desire Map*, one of my favorite writers, Danielle LaPorte, says, "You make a plan to get it … and then you pray."

All the rituals you have created thus far are your strategy; now the last thing left to do is to pray. Let me teach you how to pray and find the devotional practices that resonate most with you so you can start to feel support from and alignment with the universe and begin to deeply trust in it.

The Art of Prayer

Like a sailboat en route to a deserted island, you can set your sails, but without help you will still be floating upon a big, wild ocean with much more power than your boat. You need the universe to support you with its winds in order to take your little sailboat to the faraway islands you dream of reaching. How long it will take you to get there is ultimately not in your control. You can only set your sails; everything else is up to the universe.

When it comes to manifesting, there are so many forces of nature beyond your control. You must let go of the idea that you can control everything, including the world around you. You must trust that when the time is right, the island will appear, the anchor will drop, and you will have arrived at the place you once only dreamed about. When you believe you are powerful enough to do it all alone, you are growing your ego more than your soul, and you are actually holding yourself back.

In the sacred Hindu text the Bhagavad Gita, we are told to pray, not for the fruits of our desire, but to make an offering to the universal powers. By learning to believe you are a sacred being worthy of manifesting your dreams, you open the doors of possibility within yourself. And by trusting, asking, and praying for the universe to do the rest, you open the gates of possibility around you. This step turns the personal-growth process from an overdoing, overthinking road to burnout into a peaceful journey of surrendering and floating.

There is a Sanskrit word the yogis use for complete acceptance: *samapatti*. The nineteenth-century Hindu mystic and saint Ramakrishna advised his followers to have "total acceptance of the fact that you are a machine operated by God." If we just trust our God, our soul, our intuition, and the sacredness of our dreams, everything will work out as it should. The truth is that you can manifest anything you want in your life without struggle or stress, but with the newfound ease of simply doing what you can, then putting your hands to the sky and letting the universe do the rest.

If you aren't a religious person and find it difficult to grasp onto the concept of God, begin this step by focusing on the universal force of gravity keeping your feet grounded on this Earth and the abundance of air you breathe keeping you alive. Let these scientifically proven powers be your version of God in the beginning, and naturally you will start to feel and see the universe integrating with your entire life. The universe not only wants to see you realize your dreams; it is depending on you to.

Although I wrote this book from a place of determined willpower and soul-sent creativity, I also know that it is only the universe that can deliver it into your hands, to be read by your eyes and to make changes in your heart. Likewise, when it comes to when and how your dreams manifest in your life, the details are up to the universal powers you are praying to.

You can pray by chanting, seeing, and/or feeling. Prayer does not necessarily have to be tied to a religion; any conversation between your human existence and the soul can be considered a prayer. When you pray, a vibrational transaction moves through you, because your mind is taking a message and intentionally transmitting it as a frequency. Praying mindfully and meaningfully for exactly what you want is one way to get it.

Through the stage of dhyana, you learn to connect with whatever spirituality means to you. Because yoga is derived from the Hindu religion, I have focused most of my teachings in this chapter on the Hindu gods and goddesses, but you can practice with Jesus, Mohammad, the Buddha, or simply the force of gravity if this resonates with you. Experiment in the beginning, see what feels natural for you, and let this be your practice for connecting you to the spiritual.

The Devotional Practices

In the following section I have gathered my favorite practices for you to use to remind yourself that you are a sacred and worthy human being on a meaningful spiritual journey. I also have included practices for getting started in creating your own personal relationship with prayer. It is important to remember that the universe is supporting you and is the ultimate overseer. Equally important is believing in yourself and your worthiness to create a fantastic, inspired life for yourself. In fact, that might just be what you have been waiting for.

Chant Mantras

Japa is the practice of meditatively repeating mantras, which are divine, spiritually energetic words or phrases. Mantras can be used for many different intentions, but when we are talking about rituals for manifestation, mantras are powerful because they induce a feeling of energetic power. By repeating a sacred formula, these chants are a means of spiritual communion; they work by creating a vibrational connection between you and the universe. There are mantras for spiritual unfoldment and mantras for special powers.

Mantras work in three ways:

1. As a vibrational internal movement encouraging you to feel more deeply
2. As a form of prayer or devotion
3. To help you achieve a particular goal

While some traditional mantras are exceptionally long, I encourage you to begin your chanting practice with shorter, more personalized phrases that mean something to you.

Although there are thousands of powerful mantras you can use, here are a few simple mantras (my personal favorites) to get you started:

- **So Ham:** The simple words *So ham* translate to "I am" and sound similar to the natural sounds of the breath moving in and out.
- **Om Namah Shivaya:** This mantra is associated with qualities of prayer, divine love, grace, truth, and blissfulness. When repeated, the phrase is renowned for calming the mind and bringing spiritual insight and knowledge to the speaker. This is one of my personal favorites because it is helpful for intuitive development.
- **Om:** *Om* is believed to be the first sound that came into existence during the creation of the universe. In Hinduism, *om* (or *aum*) is the most sacred syllable, symbol, or mantra. It signifies the essence of the ultimate reality: consciousness.

You can work with mantras by saying the mantra aloud; saying the mantra quietly, to yourself; or meditating on the mantra and feeling into its vibrations. Whichever method you use, the more intention you place into your mantra practice, the more you will feel the mantras working for you.

Visit Spiritual Places

When Hindus go to a temple, they do not say, "I am going to pray" but, rather, "I am going for darshan." *Darshan* means "to see" and is the act of setting our eyes upon something that emanates the energy of a god. Your spiritual place may be as simple as an altar you create in your living room or as impressive as the Notre-Dame Cathedral. If you don't have one, start with creating an altar of meaningful objects.

In Bali, locals gather on the beach to pray to the ocean. In Hawaii, the volcanoes are believed to hold incredible sacred powers. In Sri Lanka, Buddhist devotees go to their local temple every full moon. Muslims can pray anywhere, but always face Mecca.

When you find a place that helps you believe in something bigger than yourself, stay there for a while; feel into that energy. Create spaciousness there, meditate, sense and ponder what blockages might exist within you that are keeping you from diving into the miraculous world of the unknown and her mystical ways. Then dive in fully without hesitation and experience the magical results.

Give Offerings

No matter where you go in Asia, you will see locals offering gifts of flowers, incense, money, and food to the deities, in the temples, and anywhere else they are called to offer a prayer. In India, prayer is called puja and is practiced at least once every day by nearly everyone.

By making an offering, we are asking for guidance in exchange for our devotion to honor the powers greater than us. Giving freely is how you open yourself to receiving freely. When you are trying to bring abundance into your life, the best practice is to offer what is abundant to you. Through selflessness, the ego diminishes, and the universe moves into the space where the ego once existed.

Tonglen is Tibetan for "giving and taking" or "sending and receiving." Tibetans even have a popular meditation practice called by the same name to help develop the ability to let things ebb and flow with ease. Give to honor God, and in turn God will reward you.

Study Miracles

The more you believe in miracles and magic, the more they seem to happen. If you have a highly logical mind, you might have to study the subject of miracles for a while before you start to truly believe in their existence.

The bestselling author Marianne Williamson, a leading spiritual scholar on *A Course in Miracles*, defines a miracle as "a shift in perception." Miracles are things that happen beyond our intellectual and logical understanding. Over the course of my life there have been many dreams I deemed impossible, yet eventually they happened.

Millions of stories of magic and miracles exist out there; find them and study them. A good place to start would be by reading *A Course in Miracles*. The more stories of miracles you hear, the more you understand them and believe in them, and the more you allow miracles to happen in your own life.

Stare at the Stars

Have you ever cried through an entire day only to find out, after the fact, that there was a full moon? Astrology has become one of my all-time personal favorite passions. Not only has it taught me so much about myself, but it has become an incredible tool for becoming more mindful of the present moment and growing closer to the mystical. By learning where the planets and stars were located when you were born and exploring what that means for you energetically, the energy of the cosmos will grow alive within you. When this happens, you start to understand the vastness of our interconnectedness.

Spend time watching the transitions of the stars in the present moment while also paying attention to the feelings that come over you. It won't take long before you realize that the planets, our moon, the sun, and the stars have their own unique characteristics and energies, and they very much affect the emotions, sensations, and energies happening within you.

Jyotish, a Sanskrit word meaning "the science of light," is the study of how the universe works to create beings and experiences according to one's karma. Jyotish is the ancient Vedic study of astrology and was used in a manner similar to how modern astrology is used today, for a greater understanding of who we really are, why we are really here, and why anything is here at all. The real benefit of astrology has less to do with remedies, forecasting, and gemstones and more to do with comprehending the nature of existence itself. When we stare at the stars, we begin to understand that many unknown factors play a role in our divine path, so we can trust the mysteries of life more.

Your Trust Rituals

As humans, we tend to undervalue ourselves and the importance of this journey we are on, therefore we never truly give ourselves permission to fully go after our dreams with this life. You must learn to believe and trust in yourself and your abilities if you want to create something bold with your life; otherwise you most likely will never start. If you want it to be done with ease, you must ask the universe for assistance.

If you were to perform all of the other rituals in this book and skip this one, there is a good chance you will manifest your goal, but you very well will also be building your sense of self-importance, often called your ego. As you learn how this cyclical process works, there is a good chance this will happen to you too. When we manifest our dreams without trusting in ourselves, we often become confused in who we are, lose our sense of spiritual connection, and manifest dreams only to feel more lost and confused after. You will know when this happens. Ultimately, its just better to love yourself, believe in your sacredness, and manifest as an offering to the creator, whatever that might look like for you.

You are sacred and worthy, and until you see yourself through this compassionate and loving lens, peace and happiness will have difficulties existing within you and life will be a constant chasing of worth, rather than resting in it.

The rituals you are about to create for yourself will help you realize that a soul is living within your human shell, guiding you to live and learn through this journey we call life. Your trust rituals will help you embody a newfound spiritual confidence and a trust in your soul that you have not felt before. This is how you manifest your dreams, while surrendering, relaxing, and throwing your hands (and prayers) toward the sky.

Create Your Trust Rituals: Vinyasa Krama

There are a few primary considerations to keep in mind when creating your trust rituals. Unlike the other rituals we have created, I do not feel time is an important consideration for this ritual, but more so the everyday commitment to making some form of prayer or greater appreciation happen.

Truth. First, get honest about what spirituality means to you. What is your truthful perspective of God? Do you have strong spiritual beliefs? What are they? If you do not feel like a religious/spiritual person, is there some scientific phenomena (for example gravity or the breath) that you feel you could use as your version of God to integrate these practices in your day?

Worth. When we don't honor ourselves as being sacred, it's incredibly difficult to embody a deep sense of worthiness. I believe it is the unworthiness wound living in all of us that is the entire reason we are here living these human lives. Your worth does not live in productivity and/or success – whether your career, romantic relationships, or reputation. Your worth is only increased by seeing yourself as sacred.

Are there ways your unworthiness wound is unconsciously guiding you? What do you feel makes you worthy? Do you actually believe that you are worthy to manifest your dream? What do you believe makes (or will make) you worthy? What devotional practices resonated with you the most to help you realize you are worthy?

Surrender. Are you trying to force or control your manifestation? Are you stressed and burnt out, working day and night to become or materialize something? Do you have a self-created timeline you are working on, trying to control how things work out? If so, what devotional practices can you use to surrender to the universe's divine timing? How can you put your hands in the air while still not giving up?

Support. Know exactly what you want and need and state these desires clearly. How can the universe support you? Be specific. Write it down and say it out loud.

Practice/Pray. Which of the devotional practices could you use to ask the universe to support you on a daily basis? Are you inspired to chant mantras? Visit spiritual places? Give offerings? Study miracles? Or stare at the stars? If you aren't sure, explore them all with an open mind and see what happens next.

9

The Manifestation Rituals

Consciousness itself creates the material world.

— PAM GROUT

Do you remember the childhood moment when you took your hands off the handlebars of your bike for the first time and felt the freedom and sense of accomplishment that came with your daring act? It is similar to the bliss I felt as I rode away from my first meditation intensive in the back of that pickup truck in India, my hair blowing wildly and my mind open and free. If you're a surfer, it's the sensation of successfully riding a wave after months of exhaustive trying.

That feeling of success is what comes with step eight in the yoga process: manifestation. Manifestation is the harvesting of the crops after a season of gardening. You have carefully prepared the soil of your physical body and created space. You have mindfully and consciously thought about the seed you wanted to plant and consistently pulled all the weeds that grew around it. After you did all you could do, you stopped and simply admired the way the sun and the rain amplified your efforts to make your seed grow. Now your seed has blossomed into exactly the fruit you had hoped for throughout the process.

The yogis refer to manifesting as *samadhi*. This word is derived from the root *sam-a-dha*, which means "to collect or bring together" in Sanskrit. In the final stage of yoga, you have brought together your dream (the message of your soul) with your reality (your human existence). Samadhi is the culmination of all your yogic efforts into this one moment in time.

This is the moment to stop and appreciate the hard work you put in, the inward adventure it took for you to get here, because now you have received the results. Samadhi moments are oftentimes the greatest accomplishments of your life; these are the things you dug deep for and worked hard for. Now that you are aware of and even know how to create them, they are sure to pop up more frequently in your life.

The Moment

Some dreams are obviously easier to manifest than others. But no matter how big or small your dream feels, when you do actually manifest it, it will happen in the blink of an eye. In a moment, your dream becomes your reality.

I can look back at my life and see the moments that stand out as my proudest. I think of the first yoga retreat I hosted, the moment I became a certified boat captain, the moment I made it to Cape Town after months of struggle, and the day my yoga shala in Sri Lanka opened to its first visitors. I worked long and hard for all these dreams, and then in just one moment, they happened.

When you go for that big something and you finally make it happen, you will feel contentment and a soulful satisfaction. The moment of your manifestation may feel like a reward or an accomplishment. And it should. Take time to revel in your glory. You worked hard for this. Soak in all the confidence, contentment, and satisfaction that naturally come with manifesting.

In this moment, you may feel deeply peaceful because you finally feel your connection to the sacred, the soul, and the spirit like never before. This moment is a glimpse of what enlightenment, nirvana, or liberation — whichever term resonates for you — feels like.

In the ancient yogic scriptures on samadhi, you find there are actually two types: samadhi "with seed" (*sabija samadhi*) and samadhi "without seed" (*nirbija samadhi*). When we manifest dreams of material things, such as money, or even feelings, such as happiness, this is a form of samadhi with seed. Samadhi without seed is enlightenment.

Little dreams always lead us to the bigger dreams. The more we practice manifesting samadhi with seed, the more we learn how to manifest samadhi without seed — Shangri-La, Zion, heaven, our spiritual liberation. This is ultimately the purpose of all of our work: to manifest our inner fire, our heartfelt dream.

The moment your dream becomes your reality, your soul sends you another dream. Once you take all the steps to manifest your dream, you may have epiphanies that show you how to reach the next one differently. You will constantly be changing and evolving, moving from one dream to the next. Ideally, you will continue dreaming and then manifesting over and over again, because this is how we grow our souls. In this way, dreams prove to be just a stepping-stone to the next stepping-stone.

The Cycle

Remember when that first dream you wanted to pursue seemed illogical or far-fetched? Remember in the beginning when you said you couldn't do it? Remember when you unblocked the limiting beliefs that were creating misery for so many years?

What began as a flicker of inspiration, a shooting star of an idea, has now manifested into your reality. It feels good, and it should, because your soul wants you to live through this process as a cycle, again, and again, and again. Dreams move in cycles.

With effort, we will manifest many times in our human lives; that is how we create so much spaciousness, we become open consciousness. We will develop enough mindfulness to stay focused on our truth at all times. We will hear our intuition as our first language and the thinking mind as the second. We will unblock so many of our misperceptions that the road starts to look like an open field. And we will start to see ourselves in the same power and light in which we once only saw the gods. When this happens, we liberate ourselves completely.

Once you understand how the process works, you will manifest a little more quickly the next time. You become more efficient as you grow more confident in reaching for your dreams.

As you learn, you grow. As you practice, you refine your rituals. Just as in everything else, practice makes perfect. Eventually, you start to use the eight-step yoga method for manifesting your soul's freedom.

The cycle of manifestation happens because your soul has a very big mission for you, one you are working toward, with every manifestation milestone reinforcing your belief and trust in the process. You do not need to have blind faith along this journey. Use your first manifestation to prove to yourself that the eight-step yogic system works, and then continue using it thereafter.

When it comes to understanding the concept of enlightenment, the final stage of samadhi, I believe the migration of the monarch butterfly I described in chapter 1 offers a beautiful metaphor for the yogic manifestation cycle. Like the monarch butterfly's journey, your migration might take many tries and even lifetimes, but never forget that baby steps create big results. Your own soul growth relies on the manifestation of every dream your intuition brings you in order to realize your ultimate freedom.

Spiritual growth occurs in stages, one dream at a time. Like the monarchs, you were born in this lifetime exactly where you belong to continue pursuing your spiritual evolution. As you manifest one dream, you are immediately sent on your next adventure. You may manifest hundreds of dreams in this one life and then continue in your next. Through the cycles of manifesting your dreams, you learn to unblock everything that is keeping your soul trapped within a human body. It is hard to know how long your journey will be or how many dreams it will take, but your soul is working toward something incredibly important.

The little samadhi, with seed, is practice for manifesting the big samadhi, without seed. With every dream cycle and moment of manifestation, you grow closer to the big samadhi. The big samadhi occurs when you connect your human experience with your final soulful purpose. And yoga is one of the greatest tools for spiritual evolution because it teaches you how to connect with your soul. You don't just learn how to read the road map for your journey — you actually create your own road map to liberation.

The Manifestation Rituals: Sadhana, Part 2

The Yoga Sutras state, "All powers of yoga can be attained through intuition." Your superpower is right there within you.

Your intuition not only asks you to go after particular dreams; it also shows you how. The third chapter of the Yoga Sutras, titled "Vibhuti Pada," is dedicated to explaining these superpowers. *Vibhuti* is the Sanskrit word for "power" or "manifestation." Through the steps of yoga, we acquire the power to manifest. The yogis call the manifestation process *samyama*, which combines the final three stages of yoga: unblocking, believing and trusting, and many moments of manifesting.

Patanjali says the magical superpowers you can develop from yoga are levitation, foresight, clairvoyance, the ability to see past lives, psychic awareness, and manifestation. Manifestation is available to everyone. In fact, I don't even actually believe it to be a superpower — it's just something you can develop with practice, as the yogis explained.

Now, you are ready to create one final set of rituals, the most important of all: the manifestation rituals. These are your personalized set of practices to manifest anything you want, even soul liberation.

There are moments in your life when you have it together, and there are those when you don't. In the same way that sometimes you catapult forward with momentum, you will sometimes feel held back. Know that by practicing your rituals, no matter how you feel, you are always moving in the direction of your dreams.

Create Your Manifestation Rituals: Vinyasa Krama

Begin by revisiting your dream and unblocking journaling notes. Be clear on what it is you want and then keep this intention in mind as you consider the factors below for creating your final set of rituals.

Time. Ask yourself what amount of time you can truly devote to practicing your manifestation rituals each day. Are you willing to spend longer than you have been on your ritual cycle each day, or do you need to cut out some of your previous intuition rituals to make space for other practices in the time that you've allotted?

If you have decided to minimize your intuition rituals and keep your time frame consistent, then start by revisiting each of the component parts of the previous rituals and eliminating the practices that are not as effective for you as you would like.

Spaciousness rituals. What spaciousness practices resonate most with you? Are there particular postures? Exercises? Breathing practices? Relaxation practices? Perhaps you have hobbies that you believe are helping you integrate more space into your life? Now, write these spaciousness rituals down.

Mindfulness rituals. What mindfulness practices resonate most with you? Are there particular breathing practices you can commit to each day? Now, make specific notes about how you are going to make mindfulness a daily ritual in your life.

Feeling rituals. What feeling practices resonate most with you? Yoga nidra? Chakra meditation? Long Shavasanas dedicated to feeling? Relaxation practices? Putting on jazz music and just listening within the body? In writing, specify how you are going to make a ritual of stopping whatever you're doing and focusing on feeling each and every day.

Intuition rituals. Take a look back at the practices you chose for your spaciousness, mindfulness, and feeling rituals and select a few practices from each section to create one set of practices that will become your intuition rituals.

Unblocking rituals. How will you continue acknowledging blockages and unblocking them to stay on your manifestation path? Do you have a certain affirmation that will help you unblock a limiting mindset? Can you clarify what you want by using visualizations? Are there some posture-based asana sequences you could move through to generate more confidence or perhaps more vulnerability? Do you have a daily gratitude practice? Would you benefit from one?

Would a mindset coach or life coach be beneficial for your unblocking? How about more meditative breathing? What are your daily rituals for clearing out any misperceptions and limiting beliefs? Many of these unblocking practices do not take much time; they work through consistency. I recommend making room for as many of the unblocking practices as you can commit to. Now, write down how you are going to make a ritual of unblocking and becoming each and every day.

Trust rituals. Ask yourself these questions: *Do I actually believe that I am worthy of my dream? What do I need to do to believe I am worthy? Can I trust in a universal power (or a god) to support me in my efforts? What daily practices can I use to help me believe in myself and the universe more? What daily practices can I use to remind myself that I am worthy and sacred? How can I learn to let go of control and allow the universe to support me?*

Now, create your daily rituals for reminding you that the universe is supporting you, so you can trust in it even more.

My Manifestation Rituals: An Example

Because I am so often asked, "What are your manifestation rituals?," I will share them with you, but please do keep in mind that your rituals will look a little different. My rituals make up my daily yoga practice. I take about forty-five minutes in the morning and fifteen minutes in the evening to complete this practice. When I have extra time, I will add one of the other ritual practices to my day or week. I try to practice each of the individual ritual practices — for example, my spaciousness rituals — at least once a month. For you, at this stage, the most important thing is to make sure you practice your manifestation rituals every day.

Spaciousness

1. Do at least three to five Sun Salutations (or as many as possible) daily.
2. Add postures to my asana practice as time allows. Pick postures because I am intuitively drawn to them, for unblocking and/or strengthening my manifestation.
3. Do a relaxing heart-opening pose on a yoga block for five minutes daily.

Mindfulness

1. Breathe one hundred conscious breaths daily.
2. Do the breathing practice given to me by yoga teacher O.P. Tiwari:

- ○ a.m.: Uddiyana bandha (five rounds), agni sara (five rounds), bhastrika (ten rounds), sitali (ten rounds)
- ○ p.m.: Bhramari breathing (three minutes) and trataka candle meditation (five minutes)

Feeling

1. Do a guided yoga nidra (pratyahara) meditation one time weekly.
2. Intuitively journal as often as possible.
3. Do something I love daily. Passion leads to purpose.

Unblocking

1. Visualize the moment of manifestation of my dream as often as I think of it but at least three times a week.
2. Make a gratitude list of five things every day.
3. Use affirmations every day, written around the house and said to myself.
4. Have a massage (aka relaxation) once a week.
5. Be with an intuitive community: one retreat a year.
6. Have life coach call once a month (or as needed).

Trust

1. Tell myself I am worthy of having my needs and wants met each and every day.
2. Sing mantras. (At the present moment I chant "*Om Namah Shivaya*" twenty-one times daily.)
3. Give a portion of my profits to a good cause as a part of running my soul-preneur business.

Make It Your Own

Based on the time you have allotted and the practices that resonate most with you, write out your list of manifestation rituals. Include at least one practice from each of the five stages discussed above in the "Create Your Manifestation Rituals" section:

- My rituals to create more spaciousness
- My rituals to create more mindfulness
- My rituals to create more feeling awareness
- My rituals to unblock my limiting beliefs and misperceptions
- My rituals to create belief in myself and trust in the universe

If one of these steps feels difficult, spend more time on it.

You can add a few weekly or monthly rituals as well if that feels good to you. I always try to give mindfulness a little extra love one day a week. I also try to fit in a yoga nidra practice on Sundays, because Sunday has always been a day I like to dedicate to nurturing myself with relaxation. Little weekly extras like that are totally okay!

Finally, remember the key to your practice is consistency.

Conclusion

The Connection

*It is important to expect nothing, to take every experience,
including the negative ones, as merely steps on the path,
and to proceed.*

— RAM DASS

After years of jetting around and running retreats around the world, I now found myself nestled in a small cottage hidden beneath a thick jungle on the southern coast of Sri Lanka for what would be the longest meditation intensive of my life. As the global pandemic started to change the world we were living in, my life naturally had to adjust as well. I put away work, canceled all my travel plans, and spent my days cooking, cleaning, and playing in our lush little garden with my son, Kona.

For seven weeks the Sri Lankan government did not allow us to leave the gates of our home, or we would be arrested. We were given six-hour shopping allowances once a week, which was the only time we could go out. I quit making plans for the future, as the rules and country regulations were in a constant state of flux. Day after day, I sat in the spacious emptiness of a blank to-do list. In my new unhurried reality, I started truly living in the present moment.

Just as I had in years past in Alaska, I found it was time once again to stare at the stars. As I entered the realm of seemingly endless isolation, I observed myself through the most honest lens I ever had looked through. I could see my moods and emotions — intimate, raw, and real. It was clear that I could no longer blame anything outside of myself for causing the pain and suffering I felt; all the ups and downs I was experiencing could only be coming from within, from my mind and my ego. Old childhood wounds, antiquated belief systems, and habitual tendencies — the parts of myself I often loathed — were bubbling up from deep in my subconscious to the surface of my awareness.

Slowly, with the help of my unblocking rituals, I started to surrender to these uncomfortable aspects of myself. I constantly reminded myself that pain is an essential part of our subconscious growth process. Just as there will be dreams, there will be pain the soul needs to release.

Suffering is the sandpaper grinding all the barnacles off the superficial us, leaving a pure, clear perspective of what and who we are. When you learn to relax through all the constant change happening within and outside yourself, accepting the ebb and flow of the pain and keeping your focus on your intuitive north star, you will find a simple stillness, a peace that can exist within you.

After using the yoga system to create outward accomplishments and manifestations, now I was learning to utilize that same system to embody the feelings I wanted to feel within. I wanted to feel innately worthy, peaceful, and happy most of all. By integrating the wisdom of yoga into your life in the same way I have, you will begin living more intentionally. You will come to know your truth, love and heal what you find, and then ask yourself how you want to move forward from this reality. It's a simple way to weave meaning into each day and allow yourself to learn what this life is all about along the way.

I can see how all the little intuitive messages I heard over the years guided me to where I am right now. I see how growing up in a well-populated metropolitan city led me to dream of moving into nature. While in nature, I learned how to live in a less busy way, how to sit in silence, how to study whatever bubbled up in my curiosity. I found yoga and meditation. This eventually led me to try a new career — what was once a hobby — and I became an entrepreneur. That shift gave me the privilege to be at home with my son, spending most of my days with him while also nurturing the dream within myself: to learn about myself as a spiritual being and share what I learn.

Looking back, I see my life as the thread on which I have strung a beautiful necklace from the pearls I have collected, each pearl once a dream. I am constantly living my dreams — which doesn't mean I'm constantly happy and peaceful; it just means I am finding my own path to those states through my journey of exploration. The purpose of all of this is to know myself and to be okay with who that is.

So how can you love yourself more? How can you truly start to treat yourself like the magical, soulful, intuitive human being you are? How can you make your life a purposeful collection of soul dreams? You use the rituals to get clear on what you want and to take baby steps toward that each and every day.

One of my favorite TV shows is *RuPaul's Drag Race*, a show where drag queens compete to be RuPaul's chosen favorite. Many of the show's stars share the personal hero's journey they have traveled to fully accept and love who they are — their sexual and gender orientation, what they look like, how they choose to live, the past they carry. Their stories always convey a strong message to simply love yourself just as you are, with all your wild nuances and individual uniquenesses. Each episode ends with RuPaul saying, "If you can't love yourself, how in the hell you gonna love somebody else?"

Love yourself by honoring your passions and your dreams. Love yourself by accepting that the path of exploration comes with imperfections, mistakes, and misunderstandings. Love yourself by trying new things, seeing what works and what doesn't. Love yourself by slowly evolving into your truth. Love yourself by listening to your soul, through the voice of your intuition, and becoming just that — shamelessly, vulnerably, and unapologetically. Love yourself by knowing what you need to create in your life and making it happen.

Ultimately, you are your own guru. Only you know what it is you want and need, and therefore only you can make that happen. When you make decisions from a spacious, mindful, and consciously aware place, you allow your intuition to lead you, not your ego. When you love yourself, you courageously and boldly make your dreams come true. There is no hurry to accomplish and complete your dreams; it's more important to just start integrating them into your reality however you can.

Your intuition will guide you to each wing flap of your wild and adventurous soul journey; just turn within, listen, observe, and then go with what it tells you. This process does require patience and continuous effort in order for you to achieve change, but when you make that effort, you will move toward what you want every single day. Remember that a Nepali prince became the Buddha in just thirteen years. He did that one breath at a time. He made meditation his ritual, and he found a means for eliminating his suffering and stepping into peace.

Acknowledgments

Thank you, all of you! Words can't express how grateful I am for the compassion and encouragement offered by friends and family, the precision and experience of the New World Library team, and most certainly the daily inspiration offered by my son Kona to live a life of grand adventure and purpose. Most of all, thank you to those who have taken the time to read what I have written. I wish for nothing more than peace, happiness, and health for us all. Thank you, thank you, thank you.

Endnotes

Introduction

p. 3   *"Our perception via the unconscious"*: Carl Jung, *Psychological Types* (London: Kegan Paul; New York: Harcourt, Brace, 1923), 463.

Chapter 1: The Intuitive Yogi

p. 17   *"A yogi engages himself"*: Paramahansa Yogananda, *Autobiography of a Yogi* (Kolkata: Yogoda Satsang Society of India, 2006), 224.

p. 22   *"The golden keys to unlock"*: B.K.S. Iyengar, *Light on the Yoga Sutras of Patanjali* (London: Aquarian/Thorsons, 1993), 28.

Chapter 2: Creating Space

p. 35   *"Sthira sukham asanam"*: Patanjali, Yoga Sutras 2:29, my translation.

p. 37   *"Developing such an intense sensitivity"*: B.K.S. Iyengar, *Light on Life: The Yoga Journey to Wholeness, Inner Peace, and Ultimate Freedom* (Emmaus, PA: Rodale, 2006), 29.

p. 42   *"In a special way"*: T.K.V. Desikachar, *The Heart of Yoga* (Rochester, VT: Inner Traditions / Bear & Co., 1999), 81.

Chapter 3: Becoming Mindful

p. 49   *"Rather than being your thoughts"*: Eckhart Tolle, *A New Earth: Awakening to Your Life's Purpose* (New York: Penguin, 2005), 96.

p. 65   *"'Crazy-busy' is a great armor"*: Brené Brown, quoted in Lillian Cunningham, "Exhaustion Is Not a Status Symbol," *Washington Post*, October 3, 2012,
https://www.washingtonpost.com/national/exhaustion-is-not-a-status
-symbol/2012/10/02/19d27aa8-0cba-11e2-bb5e-492c0d30bff6_story.html.

p. 77   *"You must work patiently"*: S. N. Goenka, *The Discourse Summaries* (On-
alaska, WA: Pariyatti Publishing, 2012), 18.

p. 94   *"A professional laugher"*: "The Dalai Lama: Why I Laugh," excerpt from
My Spiritual Journey, quoted in Awakin, https://www.awakin.org/read
/view.php?tid=995.

Chapter 5: Developing Awareness

p. 103   *"I have found from experience"*: Jung, *Psychological Types*, 6.

p. 105   *"The theory of relativity"*: Michele Root-Bernstein and Robert Root-
Bernstein, "Einstein on Creative Thinking: Music and the Intuitive Art of
Scientific Imagination," *Psychology Today*, March 31, 2010, https://www
.psychologytoday.com/us/blog/imagine/201003/einstein-creative-thinking
-music-and-the-intuitive-art-scientific-imagination.

p. 105   *"All great achievements of science"*: Albert Einstein, quoted in Leon
Gunther, *The Physics of Music and Color: Sound and Light* (Berlin/
Heidelberg: Springer International Publishing, 2019), 6.

p. 108   *"In my travels I spent"*: In Daniel Ladinsky, trans., *Love Poems from God:
Twelve Sacred Voices from the East and West* (New York: Penguin Compass, 2002), 249.

p. 115   *"During my seven days"*: Eben Alexander, "The Science of Heaven,"
Newsweek, November 18, 2012, https://www.newsweek.com/science
-heaven-63823.

Chapter 7: Unblocking and Becoming

p. 152   *"concentrating wholly on a single point"*: B. K. S. Iyengar, *Light on Yoga*
(New York: Schocken Books, 1979), 48.

p. 155   *"So long as they are not"*: Iyengar, *Light on Yoga*, 24.

p. 163   *"I spoke as if"*: Mother Teresa, quoted in Daniel Trotta, "Letters Reveal
Mother Teresa's Doubt about Faith," Reuters, August 25, 2007, https://
www.reuters.com/article/us-teresa-letters-idUSN2435506020070824.

p. 165   *"It is worse to stay"*: Clarissa Pinkola Estés, *Women Who Run with the Wolves* (New York: Ballantine Books, 1995), 184.

p. 170   *"Upon being harassed"*: Patanjali, Yoga Sutras 2:33, my translation.

p. 173   *Remarkably, upon his release*: Serge Schmemann, "Kasparov Beaten in Israel, by Russians," *New York Times*, October 16, 1996, https://www.nytimes.com/1996/10/16/world/kasparov-beaten-in-israel-by-russians.html.

p. 174   *"I live in the space"*: Oprah Winfrey, quoted in Owen Baxter, "7 Oprah Winfrey Quotes to Charge Your Day with Gratitude," Goalcast, July 27, 2017, https://www.goalcast.com/2017/07/27/7-oprah-winfrey-quotes-to-charge-your-day-with-gratitude/.

Chapter 8: Belief and Trust

p. 193   *"You make a plan"*: Danielle LaPorte, *The Desire Map: A Guide to Creating Goals with Soul* (Boulder, CO: Sounds True, 2014), 19.

p. 194   *"Total acceptance of the fact"*: Ramakrishna, quoted in Gregor Maehle, *Ashtanga Yoga: Practice and Philosophy* (Novato, CA: New World Library, 2011), 5.

p. 199   *"A shift in perception"*: Marianne Williamson, *The Law of Divine Compensation: On Work, Money, and Miracles* (New York: HarperCollins, 2012), 5.

Chapter 9: The Manifestation Rituals

p. 210   *"All powers of yoga"*: Patanjali, Yoga Sutras 3:33, my translation.

About the Author

Kori Hahn is a surfer, a yoga and meditation teacher, a world traveler, and a mother. When she was twenty years old, she traveled to Alaska, where she lived for twelve years in a remote cabin in close contact with nature, chopping firewood, hauling water, and skiing down towering mountains. In 2014, she founded Santosha Society, a community gathering place dedicated to nurturing more soul-fulfilling lives by integrating yoga and meditation. Through it, Hahn has hosted numerous trips around the world for hundreds of women who study Ayurveda, yoga, meditation, and all things related to soul growth, knowledge, and fulfillment. Hahn's teachings can also be found online in courses, blogs, and podcasts. When she isn't traveling, she lives in Sri Lanka with her son. Learn more at santoshasociety.com.